U0382267

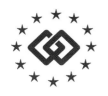

更多更好的
家庭照料服务就业

More and Better Jobs in Home-care Services

［荷兰］彼得·德克拉沃　　　　［荷兰］安伯·范德格拉夫

［荷兰］道维·格里普斯特拉　　［荷兰］贾克林·斯内德斯　著

汪消　译

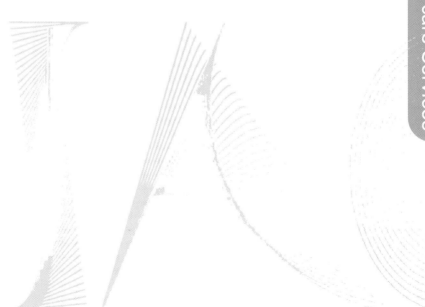

中国社会科学出版社

图字:01-2017-6199

图书在版编目(CIP)数据

更多更好的家庭照料服务就业 / (荷) 彼得·德克拉沃等著；汪消译.
—北京：中国社会科学出版社，2017.9
书名原文：More and Better Jobs in Home - care Services
ISBN 978 - 7 - 5203 - 1140 - 3

Ⅰ.①更…　Ⅱ.①彼…②汪…　Ⅲ.①老年人—家庭—护理—
服务业—研究—欧洲　Ⅳ.①R473.2②F719

中国版本图书馆 CIP 数据核字 (2017) 第 241907 号

出 版 人	赵剑英	
责任编辑	张　潜	
责任校对	胡新芳	
责任印制	王　超	

出　　版	中国社会科学出版社	
社　　址	北京鼓楼西大街甲 158 号	
邮　　编	100720	
网　　址	http://www.csspw.cn	
发 行 部	010 - 84083685	
门 市 部	010 - 84029450	
经　　销	新华书店及其他书店	

印　　刷	北京君升印刷有限公司	
装　　订	廊坊市广阳区广增装订厂	
版　　次	2017 年 9 月第 1 版	
印　　次	2017 年 9 月第 1 次印刷	

开　　本	710×1000　1/16	
印　　张	18.5	
插　　页	2	
字　　数	202 千字	
定　　价	78.00 元	

凡购买中国社会科学出版社图书,如有质量问题请与本社营销中心联系调换
电话:010 - 84083683

概　　要

　　本书探讨了为残疾和有健康问题的成人提供社区照料以及支持服务人员的招聘和留用措施。研究主要包括 10 个欧盟国家，分别是奥地利、保加利亚、丹麦、法国、德国、荷兰、波兰、葡萄牙、西班牙和英国。书中研究了上述国家的 30 个案例，分析了案例中积极的一面，即，以创造更多基于社区的成人健康与社会照护行业的就业机会，通过吸引新雇员和留住老雇员来提高工作质量。

一　政策背景

　　人口老龄化引发了长期照料岗位需求的增长。高效可行的健康与社会照料系统对欧洲社会和经济至关重要。几乎在所有欧盟成员国，健康与社会照料行业都在不断增长，该行业提供

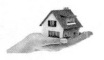

了更多的就业机会。这个行业需要更多有素质和技能的人来帮助多种慢性病患者。然而，提高这一行业的就业存在一些障碍，其中包括人员短缺，预算限制和特定的工作条件需求。要解决这些问题，在健康与社会照料行业创造强劲的劳动力并持续增长，就需要各种对策。然而，只有让从事这个行业工作的人感觉值得留在这个行业，这些政策才可持续，这就意味着，为解决照料行业劳动力短缺，制定的政策必须保证雇员有满意的工作环境和工资水平。

二　主要结论

1. 如何平衡成年残疾人社区照料和机构照料的关系因国家而异。总体来看，社区照料有一个增长的趋势。促使家庭照料发展的动力包括低成本、针对残疾人的更独立的政策、客户的偏爱以及辅助生活技术的可能性。

2. 很难确定老年人和残疾人社区照料所需劳动力的数量。只有以下几个国家有数据：奥地利有 20100 个职位，法国有 393000 个职位，荷兰有 132200 个职位，西班牙有 115900 个职位，英国有 960000 个职位。

3. 从三个国家获得的调研数据显示，家庭护工的数量在增长，奥地利平均每年增加 740 个，法国平均每年增加 19800 个，英国平均每年增加 28000 个。这一增长趋势很可能也适用于其他国家。预计这一增长趋势在未来几年将持续。

4. 总体来看，社区照料劳动力市场的特点是劳动力紧缺，尤其缺少高素质水平的劳动力。经济危机使得劳动力紧缺问题暂时得以缓解。但从长远来看，紧缺会加剧，尤其是高素质人员的紧缺会加剧。欧洲正处于经济危机的中期，危机对照料服务行业不利，因其更强调对社区照料的财政支持而不是对机构照料的支持。高失业率使得照料行业更具吸引力，对劳动力市场措施的日益重视将促进人员招募的增长。

三　劳动力市场策略

有四种劳动力市场策略已被证明可以提高行业的人员招聘和留用。

1. 确定劳动力储备的目标人群以吸引新的雇员，包括招收失业移民和流动劳动力。

2. 促进对潜在雇员的教育，例如，创造特殊的学习途径，开展活动以鼓励年轻人在这个行业选择岗位，同时改善劳动力市场与教育机构的关系。

3. 改善现有雇员的工作条件，最大限度发挥他们的潜力并将他们留在这一行业，例如，通过引入培训项目，使这一行业职业化，为已有雇员提供更多职业机会。

4. 提高组织机构的运营管理和劳动生产率，比如，运用新技术和直接支付报酬，以及在员工中更有效地分配任务。

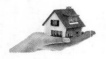

四　政策方针

1. 基于社区照料服务的招聘计划可以为外来移民提供就业机会，尤其是可以为长期失业和残疾的成年人提供就业机会。一些移民可能已经有在非正式照料机构工作的经验。获得这些目标人群需要有针对性的方法。

2. 鼓励年轻人在照料行业就业，有的放矢地针对特定人群组织活动，效果会比较好。说服男孩尤其是那些在意职业选择是否被认可的男孩从事照料行业任重道远。

3. 社会照料教育的内容和组织形式必须对学生具有吸引力，重视实践工作，如果可能，培训就安排在他们自己社区里。

4. 对已经在这个行业工作的人来说，人力资源和日常管理必须是专业的。为雇员提供实践性的培训和再培训计划，可以提高照料行业的标准。培训地点离家近、尽可能免费并将培训安排在上班时间，实施小班培训，效果会更理想。

5. 辅助技术为这一领域提供了很大的潜力。需要培训雇员学会使用这些技术。让客户和提供服务的人都接受这些技术也是很重要的。

6. 需要特别关注的是可持续性，尤其是资助项目。这就是说，公共基金资助的项目要有稳定的经费，要有效协调资金安全运行，并且有一个单位或组织担任领导角色。

7. 把成功的方案移植到别的地区、国家或部门时需要有周密的计划，这样才能把成功的新方法纳入常规行动和政策。这可能包括使用欧盟基金进行跨国合作。

8. 具有解决家庭照料和社区照料的劳动力市场问题的政治意愿，是实现成功、可持续和可转化措施的重要先决条件。目前，政策和政治承诺之间存在差距。虽已立法，但今后家庭照料劳动力市场的发展还需要持续的政治支持。

9. 对于欧盟及其成员国来说，政治支持是为招聘和留用措施提供结构性基金所必需的。

10. 数据的收集和统计使用可以不断完善，为各国和欧盟当局发展、监测、评估和调整相关劳动力市场政策提供依据。

目　　录

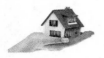

引　言

一　政策背景

2013 年 2 月，欧盟委员会在它的"社会投资一揽子计划"里号召成员国优先考虑社会事业投资并实现福利的现代化，以此来应对它们所面临的重大挑战。这些挑战包括严重的金融危机、加剧的贫困和社会排斥以及年轻人中创纪录的失业率。除此之外，还要加上人口老龄化和劳动年龄人口减少的挑战，这些都考验着国家社会事业系统的可持续性和妥善性（欧盟委员会，2013b）。

在委员会职员工作文件"老龄化社会的长期照料——挑战和政策权衡"中，"社会投资一揽子计划"指出了要特别关注长期照料问题。文件陈述了可以通过预防、康复和创造更多的适老环境，以及开发更多提供照料的有效途径，来减少对长期

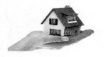

照料的需求。

　　拥有一个可以提供健康和社会照料的、有效运转和高质量的系统对欧盟社会和经济来说至关重要。身体健康情况不佳会造成社会排斥和参与社会活动的障碍。与此同时，健康和社会照料行业正快速发展，提供了更多"白色工作"的机会。① 人口老龄化的增长需要高质量的照料，这一行业仍有更多扩大就业的潜力。然而，在欧盟 2012 年的"向着高就业复苏"信息里，欧盟委员会确定了在这一行业创造就业的若干障碍问题（欧盟委员会，2012b）。包括：缺少新雇员来代替退休的雇员；需要出现新的健康照料方式以应对多种慢性疾病；预算限制；需要少量工作条件补偿金。

　　为克服上述问题和支持健康与照料行业创造强劲增长的劳动力，一些国家正采取不同措施来改善状况，另一些国家可以从中吸取经验教训。

二　研究目的

　　本研究的主要目的是探讨如何在照料行业创造就业机会（包括招聘和留用）。尤其是探讨如何为有身体、智力残疾，慢性疾病或有精神健康问题的成人提供家庭和社区照料以及支持

---

　　① 介绍目前欧盟委员会的当务之急时，主席巴罗佐强调根本需求是创造就业机会，对欧洲来说尤其是"绿色工作"（与环境和气候变化管理有关的行业）和"白色工作"（健康与社会服务）的机会。

服务。研究描述了入选成员国的现状，并提出了对提高照料行业劳动力的规模和素质都有效的措施。

为达到这一主要目的，本研究设定了以下具体目标。

（1）确定 10 个欧盟成员国，提高家庭照料雇员的规模和素质，降低雇员流动率，制定政策和法规促进照料行业劳动力增长；

（2）对入选国的家庭照料和社区照料劳动力市场现状进行描述；

（3）对入选国如何贯彻不同的聘用和留用措施以及取得的成效进行记录。

三　概念界定

本研究的重点是关于残疾人家庭照料和社区照料的就业问题。社区照料的定义是，为人们提供健康和社会照料使得他们能生活在社区里。[①] 而机构照料是指由寄宿机构提供的照料。已有的一些资料可以明显区分家庭照料（代替社区照料）和机构照料。[②]

然而，在有些国家，术语"家庭照料"的意义很狭窄。因

[①] 社区照料和个人与家庭服务（PHS）有部分重叠。PHS 的定义泛指在家里为家庭及成员提供健康服务活动：照顾儿童、长期照料老人和残疾人、辅导班、家庭维修、园艺工作、信息通信技术支持和福利工作（见欧盟委员会，2012b）。

[②] 例如，Rodrigues 等，2012。这里家庭照料的定义是经过正式的需求评估后由专业人员在家里提供的照料。"照料"的意思是家庭救助服务、个人照料和支持、技术和康复照料。

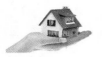

此，术语"社区照料"被优先使用，与此同时，涉及的工作人员仍被称为"家庭照料工"，这样可以更准确地描述他们的工作，而不是使用术语"社区照料工"。

在本研究里，家庭照料工被定义为提供以下健康和社会照料的人员。

（1）为特定目标人群（身体或智力残疾的成年人，有慢性疾病或精神健康问题，尤其是不到退休年龄的人）提供健康和社会照料服务；

（2）提供特定的照料形式（长期照料）；

（3）在特定的场所工作（社区照料，区别于机构照料）；

（4）正式的有报酬的工作（区别于非正式、无报酬照料）。

这一定义显示，我们的讨论不是针对某一特定的职业或专业。一个专业对自己的定义通常通过特定的专业特性、专业历史或自有组织。一个职业的定义通常是某些人需要具备进入这一行业劳动力市场的任职资格并且在职业生涯中不断实践。对职业和专业的定义因国家不同而有相当大的差异（参见 Cede-fop，2012）。

因此本研究关注的是上述劳动力市场的活动形式和目标。基于这些活动，本研究的重点是一些对应的职业人群，大致与NACE编码88.10一致（指为老年人和残疾人提供没有住所的社会服务，包括家庭护工、社会照料工人、社工、活动工作人员[①]、社区护

[①] 帮助人们从事社区活动或帮助人们重新找到工作的工作人员。

士以及其他专业人员，如治疗师）。某些初级医疗保健职业人群，家庭医生、牙医不包括在内。

四　成员国的选择

本报告深入研究了 10 个欧盟成员国，国家的选择基于以下标准。

（1）地理位置：来自欧洲所有四个区域的国家（北欧、东欧、南欧和西欧）；

（2）加入欧盟的时间：来自加入欧盟时间不同的国家，分别是来自 2004 年欧盟扩大之前的 15 个成员国，2004 年入盟国家和 2007 年入盟国家；

（3）非机构化程度：家庭照料和社区照料比例低和比例高的国家；

（4）已有的相关政策、法规和议案：家庭照料工人缺乏的问题已经凸显，并有相关政策、法律和议案用以增加雇佣的国家。

基于这些指标，暂时选择了 10 个国家。为了对问题的种类、政策途径和可能的有趣案例有一个第一印象，从而进行深入研究，入选国的专家进行了案头调查。他们对该领域的一般主题和发展进行了调查，也确定了一些以解决问题为目的的议案个例。

这一行业的特征在各国都是相似的，一个国家的经济和政

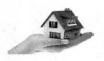

策背景（例如从一般政策、法规、集权程度、正式对非正式照料以及基金结构的角度来说）决定了这些问题的讨论方式，以及从政策、条例和举措上做何反应。

最后选定的 10 个成员国如下：奥地利、保加利亚、丹麦、法国、德国、荷兰、波兰、葡萄牙、西班牙和英国。

五　研究内容

首先，作为研究方法，本研究使用了三个模型。

（1）劳动力市场模型，规划了现在和预期的劳动力市场供需情况以及劳动力市场供需差异造成的问题。

（2）PESTLE 分析模型，分析了政治、经济、社会、技术、法律和环境因素对劳动力市场的影响。

（3）解决方案模型，对解决劳动力市场问题的方法进行了分类。

这三个模型（详见附录1）形成了制订研究问题、收集和分析数据以及完成报告的基础。

本研究始于对相关欧盟政策和统计的案头研究。

其次，在每一个入选国，来自欧盟社会和经济研究网（ENSR）的各国专家收集了相关国家的信息（专家姓名和组织详见附录2）。通过使用固定的模板，使得用结构化的方式收集国家信息成为可能。

各国专家撰写了格式相似的国家报告，便于比较和得出结论。综合而言，主题有：①政策和举措发展的背景以及要解决的问题；②政治和法律框架；③结构框架和基金结构；④招聘和留用雇员的项目类型。

另外，各国专家对家庭照料领域创造和保留就业的 30 个成功案例进行了研究。典型案例被选出来分别代表 4 种解决这个行业劳动力市场问题的策略：①以劳动力市场储备为目标；②促进和推动潜在雇员的教育；③改善现有雇员的工作环境；④改善组织的运行管理和劳动生产率。

最重要的筛选标准是这个方法必须既有创新性又有实用性。任何一个既创新又实用的方法可以被定义为以下项目、政策或解决方法。

（1）提高工作人员数量、质量或者降低雇员离职率的努力尝试。

（2）以有身体或智力残疾的人，有慢性疾病或精神健康问题的成年人，以及提供社区照料服务的工作人员为特定目标。

（3）解决照料工人劳动力市场特殊的数量和质量供需不符以及缺乏透明度的问题。

（4）采用上述 3 种策略中的一个或多个以防止劳动力市场供需不符。

（5）具有清晰和发展的眼光与方法。

（6）具有适合方法运用的条件。

（7）遵从并认真记录程序和步骤。

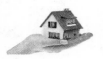

（8）从达到目标的人群、后续工作、内在和外在影响的角度来说，已被证明是成功的，至少被评估过一次并且效果显著的方法。

除了创新性和实用性，这些措施还必须有大量的外展服务、雇员和基金。针对每一种策略，选择了各种各样的方法。综合结果选择的案例被认为是关于招聘和留用雇员措施和方法方面高质量和可转让的典范，对所有欧盟成员国的政策制定者是受益的。

总之，每一个案例研究包括 5 部分。

（1）问题定义：要解决特定的劳动力市场什么问题？

（2）方法：解决这个问题使用了什么方法？这个方法的要素是什么？

（3）背景因素：哪些条件影响了实践效果？哪些因素促进了措施的成功？

（4）结果：这个措施结果如何？创造了多少就业机会？问题解决了吗？

（5）学到的经验：直接相关的或其他机构从这个特定的措施里学到了什么？主要的成功和失败的因素是什么？此措施可持续性如何？这个方法多大程度可转换并用于其他情况？

在对这 30 个案例进行分析研究的基础上，才可能对成功和潜在失败的因素进行总结，明确招聘和留用措施的可持续性和可转换性，形成创造就业的政策建议。

六　报告结构

第一章记述了欧洲健康和社会照料行业的欧盟政策背景和当前支出统计，照料对象以及行业就业情况。第二章记述了这一劳动力市场的特点和影响它的背景因素。第三章综述了30个案例中对行业招聘和留用有益的实践，并将它们按各自举证的劳动力市场策略进行分类。第四章总结了各项措施的效果以及它们对就业的影响。第五章讨论了措施中与成功和失败有关的因素。第六章得出了一些研究结论并给出了一系列政策建议。

报告最后的附录由研究的分析框架和这个研究项目相关的各国专家的概述组成。10个国家的研究包括案例研究将在另外的报告里陈述。

第一章　欧洲的健康与社会照料政策和统计数据

　　本章开篇讲述的是健康和社会照料行业相关的欧盟政策要点。与近期的"社会投资计划"关系尤为密切，它敦促成员国优先考虑社会投资并实现福利制度的现代化。讨论部分则总结了今后欧盟卫生领域劳动力需求的政策，主要聚焦于五个方面：劳动力规划、预期所需技能、培训和流动、招聘和留用以及欧盟基金。本章还提供了关于残疾或有健康问题成年人的照料和支持服务劳动力市场的欧盟统计资料。

一　欧盟政策

（一）欧洲 2020

　　"欧洲 2020"是欧盟委员会于 2010 年 3 月 3 日提出的一个关于欧盟经济提升的十年行动计划。这个行动计划的目标是使各国和欧盟政策更加协调，实现"智能、可持续、包容性增长"（欧盟委员会，2010b）。

社会保障委员会2011年的一个报告分析了"欧洲2020"计划的社会层面，传达了十个关键信息。其中一个关键信息是提高健康照料和长期照料的有效性、可持续性和响应能力（欧盟委员会，2011）。

欧盟通过开放合作方式①促进各国间的长期照料合作，重点关注途径、质量和可持续性。关于这个报告，与上述三个方面最密切相关的目标如下。

（1）提高所有人口层次长期照料服务的供给（家庭、社区和机构服务的组合）。

（2）降低有效性照料和质量的地域差异。

（3）优先考虑量身定制的照料和支持服务，以确保人们可以尽可能久地生活在家里；无法获得这样服务的地方，在机构照料方面做出类似的适应性改进。

（4）建立质量保证对策。

（5）把重点放在所有年龄段人的健康提升上，包括老年、疾病预防和康复政策。

（6）通过正规的雇员培训、激励机制和工作条件来保证充足的人力资源。

---

① 开放合作方式（OMC）是成员国之间合作的一个框架。OMC的成果具有潜在的约束性特征，它实际上是"软法律"——依赖于同伴的压力。

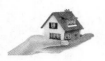

　　另一个解决健康和照料行业预期的劳动力短缺的重要方式是"促进和推动欧盟内部劳动力的流动，并从结构基金角度使得劳动力的供需与拨出的财政支持更匹配"（欧盟委员会，2010b，p. 18）。为此，欧盟已经采取了几个具体的行动以改进长期照料行业的劳动力短缺问题。

　　（二）就业计划

　　"就业计划"（2012 年 4 月发布）是一系列政策文件，检查了欧盟就业政策如何与其他一些政策领域产生交集以支持其智能、可持续和包容性增长（欧盟委员会，2012d）。它确定了欧盟能提供最大就业潜力的领域，以及欧盟国家创造更多就业机会的最有效的途径。

　　由于健康和社会照料行业具有很高的就业潜力，"就业计划"对"白色工作"给予了特别关注，并且它包括了一个欧盟健康劳动力的行动计划。实施该计划的目的是促进欧盟合作并分享好的实践经验，从而改进健康劳动力计划和预测，提前考虑今后需要的技能以及改善健康领域专业人员的招聘和留用，同时减少移居对卫生系统造成的不利影响。

　　作为就业计划的一部分，委员会也发布了一个开发个人与家庭服务潜力的雇员工作文件（欧盟委员会，2012b）。这个计划的目的是针对以下几方面明确对策。

　　（1）通过将过多的日常家务工作移交给提供服务的人员，包括儿童和老人的照料，以实现更好的"工作—生活"平衡。

（2）为技术含量相对较低的，尤其是家政服务创造就业机会。

（3）提高照料的质量。

经过与投资人（包括国家主管部门、社会合伙人以及服务的使用者和提供者）的磋商，将进一步发展这些行动计划。

（三）社会投资计划

"社会投资计划"（2013）陈述了成员国和委员会的欧盟政策框架以及将采取的具体行动，在计划指导下使用欧盟基金进行改革，社会保障系统将更高效和有效。

社会投资计划的一个重要组成部分是委员会雇员工作文件，即"老龄化社会的长期照料——挑战和政策选择"（欧盟委员会，2013a）。它认为欧洲需要做好准备，到2060年，需要长期照料的年龄段人群（80岁及以上的人）可能将增至现在的三倍。从这一重要人口变化的角度来看，目前对老年人长期照料需求的应对方式是不可持续的。文件强调了应对这一挑战的方法，可以通过疾病预防、康复以及创造更多适合高龄老人的环境来降低长期照料需求，同时开发更多提供照料的有效途径。

通过开发新的途径缩小长期照料需求与供给的差距，欧盟在促进这一领域的创新和提高社会投资上可以发挥重要作用，例如，欧洲创新合作伙伴的"积极健康老龄化与居家辅助项目"。欧盟也可以用结构基金推动高龄和谐环境和优质专业照

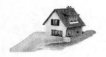

料的投资。

为了防范长期照料的风险，欧盟的经济政策和社会保障委员会将持续对社保的经济可持续性和充足的社会保障进行监督。这对于实现"欧洲2020"计划中设定的一系列目标起到决定性作用——健全的公共财政，高就业水平和减少贫困。

委员会关于长期照料的文件建议成员国对社会投资计划给予特别的关注，结合健康防护措施、积极老龄化措施以及生产力驱动的照料服务，以提高老年人继续独立生活的能力，哪怕他们变得虚弱或残疾。此外，通过各国的政策建议，欧盟的政策导向已越来越多地优先考虑公共支出的质量，关注这个领域支出的有效性的提高，从而确保即使在人口老龄化的形势下，社会保障也能恰当地应对长期照料的危机。

二　政策行动

成员国认同健康和社会照料行业的挑战，因此，在2010年12月的EPSCO（就业、社会政策、健康和消费者事务理事会）会议上，成员国邀请欧盟委员会协助处理健康劳动力的长期问题。下面一节讨论了欧盟近几年采取的几项行动和措施。这些行动围绕五个关键问题进行了分类：劳动力规划、技能预期、培训和劳动力流动、招聘和留用实践以及通过欧盟结构基金提供经费。

（一）劳动力规划

委员会认为，健康行业劳动力规划是当今欧洲面临的最大挑战之一。目前，缺乏可比较的统计数据使得预测不可靠。因此，一个"健康劳动力规划和预测欧盟联合行动（2013—2015）"正在实施。为确保在欧盟层面上采取的行动可以支持劳动力规划，在对策研究上，委员会指出，欧盟必须支持创造通用的定义、指标、举措和方法，并且与数据收集机构密切合作，例如，欧盟统计局，经济合作与发展组织（OECD）以及世界卫生组织（Matrix Insight，2012）。"卫生劳动力规划欧洲观测台"（2008年卫生劳动力绿皮书之后创建）担任协调员的角色。行动项目的目标是提供可比较的统计数据以及新的可靠的预测模型。在制订健康照料工人的教育、培训、工作条件和招聘的政策干预方面，预测将发挥重要作用。

（二）技能预期

第二个挑战是明确长期照料工人需要具备的技能。将照料从机构转移到家庭，对新技术的运用和不同诊断技术的运用都会对今后相关技能产生影响。欧盟开展了几个项目以规划健康照料行业的技能：一个正在调查照料和保健劳动力就业和技能的欧洲部门委员会的可行性，另一个是健康护理助手试验网络，正在付诸实施。这两个项目将有助于形成欧盟技能的全貌，对需要的新兴技能进行了概述，并包含了一个通用的职业

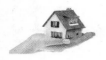

和技能的多语言分类。来自 Cedefop（欧洲职业培训发展中心）的技能预测将是技能全貌的另一个构成要素。

（三）培训和劳动力流动

第三个挑战关注的是为人们提供恰当的培训以避免岗位需求与教育不匹配。2012 年 8 月，欧盟倡议建立一个试验性质的健康照料行业的"行业技能联盟"。这个联盟汇聚了教育供应商、行业专家（例如行业联合会）以及公立和私立教育主管部门，以创建新的课程和培训方法，为学生提供劳动力市场需要的技能。2012—2014 年 "Erasmus for All"（全民伊拉斯谟）计划是欧盟的一个提高跨境教育的基金项目，也适用于健康照料从业人员，两个政策都是依据"终身学习计划"及其持续专业发展的承诺。欧盟委员会在专业资格证书的一项规定中阐明，成员国需要相互承认专业资格证书。这样做的目的是提高健康照料工人的积极性和专业技能，同时提高劳动力的跨境流动。流动和移居被认为很重要，因为劳动力市场的短缺也是跨地域的。

（四）招聘和留用实践

医院和健康照料行业的欧洲社会对话在人员招聘和留用实践的知识共享方面发挥了重要作用。在这个对话里，欧洲公共服务工会联合会（EPSU）、欧洲医院、健康照料雇主协会（HOSPEEM）制订指导方针、标准和最佳实践。举例来

说，这就形成了 2010 年招聘和留用行动的框架和跨境招聘的
行为准则。

（五）欧盟结构基金资助

欧盟通过分配欧盟结构基金的方式直接参与健康与照料行
业的改进工作。欧盟委员会在 2012 年欧洲健康劳动力行动计
划里阐明"成员国被敦促最大限度地使用欧洲资金调度工具，
以支持解决健康照料行业劳动力短缺以及促进创造就业的行
动"（欧盟，2012a，p. 12）。

两个关系最密切的基金是欧洲社会基金（ESF）和欧洲地
区发展基金（ERDF）。ERDF 可以促进照料行业基础设施和更
多技术因素的发展（例如，建设一个社区照料中心），而 ESF
主要关注的是培养技术优良的人员和提高社会包容度。最近被
采用的 ESF 2014—2020 条例就更加重视就业、劳动力流动和终
身学习。这可能意味着更多的资金将被分配到照料行业用于创
造就业和留用人员。

"机构照料过渡到社区照料特设专家组"主张提高社区照
料的投资。在 2012 年关于健康的老龄化的信息交流中，欧盟
委员会强调当务之急是从机构照料转变为社区照料，同时，增
强被照料人的独立生活能力（欧盟委员会，2012c，p. 11），在
残疾计划里也提到了这一点。

总之，欧盟没有命令在健康与社会照料以及就业领域强制
执行这些规则。然而，它对改进健康与照料行业的可获得性、

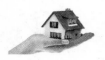

可持续性和质量给予了强有力的承诺，要实现上述目标主要依靠合作和目标设定。欧盟的目标近来变成了具体的试点项目，即，调研整个健康与社会照料行业（尤其是老龄人群的长期照料）怎样才能被一个繁荣、积极和专业合格的从业人员群体所支持。另外，欧盟欢迎改进健康与社会照料行业的投资建议。

三　欧盟统计数据

欧盟范围内健康与社会照料服务行业的统计数据很多。然而，这些统计有两方面的局限性。一是许多统计没有区分机构照料、家庭照料及社区照料；二是绝大多数长期照料的统计没有区分不同年龄人群的服务（儿童、未达到退休年龄的成年人以及达到退休年龄的老人）。因此，在解读本节关于支出、受众和就业的统计数据时要考虑到这些局限性。[①]

（一）支出

根据 2012 年老龄化报告，2012 年欧盟 27 国的长期照料支出占 GDP 的 1.8%（欧盟委员会，2012e）。报告指出，欧盟国家长期照料支出因国家不同而有很大差异：荷兰的长期照料支出占 GDP 的 3.8%，奥地利为 1.2%，爱沙尼亚只有 0.8%。虽

---

① 涉及有关健康与社会照料服务统计局限性的资料来源包括 Huber，2007；欧盟委员会，2006；以及"欧洲健康、老龄化和退休调查"研究（www.share-project.org/），2012。

然大多数人获得的是基于家庭背景的照料，但是这一类型照料只反映了支出的30%—50%，这意味着家庭照料支出大约相当于欧盟27国GDP的0.6%—0.9%（Rodrigues等，2012）。还必须注意，涉及这一特定照料类型，不同国家间有很大的差异（图1）。

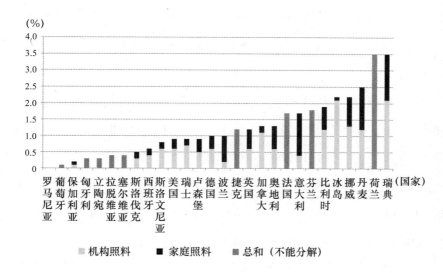

图1　欧洲和北美洲2009年或最近一年不同照料场所的长期照料公共支出（占GDP的百分比）

注："总和"表示无法获得照料场所的可靠信息。图中没有考虑照料的私人支出，这一定程度解释了国家排序的出乎意料（例如，美国排在了低支出国家里）。

来源：Rodrigues等，2012。

（二）长期照料的受众

2008年OECD（经济合作与发展组织）国家平均2.3%的人口使用了正规的长期照料服务。五分之一被照料人的年龄在

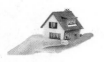

64 岁及以下。估计 65 岁以下的人只有 1% 享有某种长期照料。超过半数的长期照料是由家庭或社区照料场所提供的，根据2011 年"健康一览和招聘员工"的报告（经济合作与发展组织，2011a，2011b），平均来看，退休年龄以下的被照料人数比例高于退休年龄以上的。不同国家使用正规长期照料服务的人口数量差别很大，从波兰的占人口的 0.2% 到奥地利的 5.1%。经济合作与发展组织估计，80% 的家庭照料提供给了 65 岁以上的人。

由于明显的去机构化照料的趋势，以及老龄化和非正规照料的减少，导致家庭照料需求的增加，预计到 2050 年，家庭照料的人数将增加 130%（欧盟委员会，2006）。社区照料的趋势也反映了这样的事实，在 2007 年欧盟关于卫生和长期照料的特别民意调查中，绝大多数的调查对象都声明他们更喜欢社区照料而不是机构照料（欧盟委员会，2007）。因此，社区照料与不到退休年龄就接受长期照料的成人关系密切，尽管这一群体的绝对数量不大。

（三）劳动力需求

经济合作与发展组织估计，长期照料是健康与社会照料行业增长最快的部门（经济合作与发展组织，2011b）。它预计到2050 年，从事长期照料工作的人数将是现在的两倍。这一增长是受需要照料的老年人数量的增加以及非正式照料的减少所驱动的（欧盟委员会，2012e）。其他促进需求增长的因素包括疾病谱变化以及对照料和生活质量的态度与期望值的变化。很遗憾，没有不同种类照料长期劳动力结构的分解统计数据。乐观的估算来自经济合作与发展组织用于长期照料的受众，他们表明这个行业大约80%的工作人员从事的是老人的照料工作。

家庭照料和社区照料服务从一个方面为老人和残疾人提供了经济上可持续的照料与支持方式。这些服务类型在欧盟已经比较普遍。根据欧盟统计局2010年的数据，个人服务与家庭照料服务有部分重叠——代表了欧盟540万个工作职位，这一数字今后还会增加以应对需求的增长（Andor，2011）。

第二章　劳动力市场背景

　　本章描述了为残疾或有健康问题的成人提供照料与支持服务的行业人员招聘背景，以及留用措施的产生与执行。它基于大量欧洲近期的出版物，以及 10 个国家的专家关于这方面的研究报告提供的信息。主题包括家庭照料占总照料的份额，劳动力市场的特点以及影响照料与支持服务劳动力市场就业的客观因素。

一　家庭照料与机构照料

　　为残疾的成人提供长期家庭照料和机构照料的比例因国家而异。图 2 说明了 65 岁及以上人群的比例（通常，65 岁以下残疾人照料和支持服务的这一比例低于 65 岁及以上人群）。

　　不管国家间的差异如何，对各国的研究分析清楚地表明，

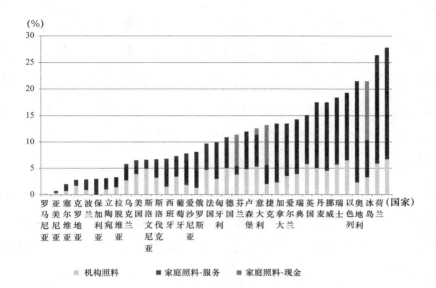

图2　65 岁及以上人获得机构照料、国家提供的家庭照料或现金

购买的照料服务的百分比（2009 年或最近一年）

注：比利时、奥地利的数据是 60 岁以上的；法国是 60 岁以上家庭照料的。一些国家的原始数据在涉及年龄组时和 65 岁以上这一截止点不一致。"家庭照料服务"包括那些现金购买和国家提供服务组合的。为避免重复计算，对意大利"家庭照料—现金"部分的估计是保守的估算。卢森堡和德国的分解数据是从总受益人里推断的。照料的自费支出没有考虑，没有对一些国家老龄人口比另一些国家多这一人口统计学的因素进行修正。

来源：Rodrigues 等，2012。

欧洲国家总的偏好是非机构照料而不是机构照料。总之，欧洲国家的社会和政治气候都赞同家庭照料。

提供更多非机构照料的一个原因是降低费用，这是需求增长和经济危机共同驱动的。通常，政府认为家庭照料和社区照

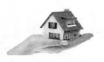

料比机构照料便宜，因其无须提供住房或场地的费用，运营成本低，邻里和家庭成员也会提供更多的帮助。然而，去客户的家里会有相关的费用，尽管这些费用可以通过信息与通信技术以及家庭照料在地区层面更好地组织来降低。

政府提高家庭照料水平的另一个原因是让患者可以尽可能长久地在他们自己的环境里独立生活和行动。最近"欧洲家庭照料"报告显示，客户通常更喜欢家庭照料而不是机构照料（Genet 等，2012）。斯洛文尼亚是一个例外，那里被抚养的老人更喜欢机构照料。不知道这一不同喜好的原因是什么，进一步的研究会阐明斯洛文尼亚的特殊情况。

另外，辅助生活技术的发展使得家庭照料变得更加可行。

二 劳动力市场特征

在这个研究里，运用了附录1的劳动力市场模型来表示家庭照料和社区照料劳动力市场的供需差异。根据已有数据，这部分首先尽可能描述了劳动力市场的大小（需方）。然后，详尽表述了劳动力市场需方和供方的差异。

（一）照料就业范围

总体来说已有的家庭和社区照料信息是分散的，只有部分可比性。本研究包括的一些国家有行业代码为 88.10（服务于老年人和残疾人的不提供住宿的社会工作活动）的数据。除了行业代码88.10的数字，一些国家的专家还提供了更高聚合等级的就业数字。表1概括了已有数据。

表1

国家	NACE（行业代码）88.10的就业情况	其他相关就业数字
奥地利	2012年，20095个雇员；（与2008年17140个雇员相比）平均每年增长740个	除了专业人员，平均9300人从事义务的民间服务（部分是社会照料）
保加利亚	没有NACE88.10数据	2011年从事人类卫生与社会工作的雇员总数是153500人，2006年是122513人 2011年家庭照料和社会工作雇员是28075人（2009年是27990人）
丹麦	没有NACE88.10数据	2011年健康与社会照料工人和助手[a]总数是122918人，2008年是119644人
法国	2010年，393700个雇员，其中社区工作261400人（NACE88.10A），就业支持工作122100人（NACE88.10C）。数字在增加，与2008年相比，社区支持工作增加了16%（NACE88.10A），就业支持工作增加了3%（NACE88.10C）；NACE88.10A与NACE88.10C合计年平均增加19800人	家庭照料服务的工作小时数相当于42900个每周工作35小时的全职工作（法国合法的每周工作时间）。这些小时绝大多数相当于家庭帮助小时，被分类在NACE97.00"作为家政人员雇主的家务活动"
德国	没有NACE88.10数据	至2009年年底，代表社会长期照料保险计划提供正规照料（带工资的）的雇员总数是890283人，其中268900人在家庭照料和社区照料领域工作
荷兰	粗略估计，2012年有2055个单位雇用了132300个雇员[b]	2011年，健康和社会照料行业总的工作职位是1348900个。精神病患者照料、残疾人照料、家庭照料服务和福利服务各分支分别占88000个、161000个、193000个和72000个职位（总共514000个职位）

更多更好的家庭照料服务就业

续表

国家	NACE（行业代码）88.10 的就业情况	其他相关就业数字
波兰	没有 NACE88.10 数据	2011 年总共大约 650000 人被卫生与社会照料相关行业雇佣[c] 没有提供长期健康照料的人员的具体数字。2011 年大约 7000 人在社会援助中心提供社会照料（一般照料服务和特殊照料服务）[d]
葡萄牙	没有 NACE88.10 数据	2010 年有 6100 个私营设施或服务机构提供社会照料（NACE87 和 88 分别是居家照料和社会照料），营利性和非营利性兼有，雇用了 114900 人（其中 61800 人从事居家照料，53100 人从事社会照料）。2008 年雇用了大约 113200 人（其中 59200 人从事居家照料，54000 人从事社会照料）
西班牙	2012 年有 2489 个机构 115900 个雇员（2009 年有 2348 个机构 102300 个雇员）	
英国	2009 年英国有 4720 个注册公司（公立的、营利的以及志愿的/慈善的）大约 960000 个雇员（比 2008 年增加了 3%，比 2005 年增加了 9%）；基于 2008—2009 年的数据，年均增加 28000 个	英格兰仅 2011 年估计有 185 万个成人社会照料职位（比 2010 年增加 4.5%），而成人社会照料的实际劳动力数量只有 163 万个 家庭照料和非家庭照料分别占 48% 和 52%。大多数社会照料职位（65%）由独立雇主提供，其次是直接付费的被照料人（23%），地方政府（9%）以及英国国家医疗服务体系（约 4%）

注：a 执业包括护士、理疗师、职业治疗师、老师/教育工作者、社会教育家、心理学家、社工、社会教育家助理、社会与健康照料工人、社会与健康照料/教育助理、社会与卫生助理。

b 这是作者根据荷兰中央统计办公室关于 NACE88.10 机构与雇员以及雇员分类的数据做的粗略估计。估计如下：最少—18900 个雇员；居中—39585 个雇员；最多—132270 个雇员。

c 根据国际标准职业分类，与健康和社会照料相关的职业数量如下：513 个个人照料和相关工人，223 个照料和助产辅助专业人员，323 个照料和助产辅助专业人员以及 913 个家庭和相关助手、清洁工人和洗衣工人。

d 这只代表提供长期社会照料服务劳动力的一部分，因为在被照料人家里的社会照料服务被市政当局的社会援助中心分包给了私人公司。这些公司雇员的数量没有收集。

来源：信息由各国专家提供。

26

尽管数据不完整而且只有部分具有可比性，国家报告清楚地描述了家庭照料工人数量增长的总体情况，但是是在残疾成年人照料这一特殊领域。

欧洲家庭照料报告证实了这一领域仍然缺乏数据的情况。符合这个综述的需要的家庭照料工人数量的数据无法广泛获得（Genet 等，2012）。

（二）劳动力供需的差异

总体来说，家庭照料劳动力市场的形势是不利的。

首先，数量上有差异。欧洲家庭照料报告指出了以下几个国家雇员的总体紧缺：奥地利、比利时、保加利亚、塞浦路斯、捷克、芬兰、法国、希腊、立陶宛、葡萄牙和斯洛文尼亚（Genet 等，2012）。

其次，素质有差异。在同一个研究领域里，一些国家——保加利亚、塞浦路斯、丹麦、爱沙尼亚、法国、德国、希腊、卢森堡和挪威——报告了缺乏足够合格的家庭照料职员。例如，比利时和保加利亚居家照料助手太少，而法国、希腊、立陶宛和斯洛文尼亚通常家庭照料专业人员太少。

从照料工人的角度来看，有质量上的差异。总体来看，工作质量（报酬和其他劳动待遇、工作环境和工作时间）比其他行业低：家庭照料是一项费力的工作，有些护理人员有一个以上的雇主，一天要为两个或更多的人服务，工作时间也是一个

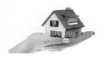

问题。不管怎样，有些欧洲国家通过社会伙伴的集体协议已经开始改善工作质量。

这一行业还存在行业形象问题，部分由于客观因素（劳动待遇和工作环境），部分由于主观因素（负面的看法和公众的意见）。总之，形象问题将持续存在，难以防止。

除了这些概貌，各国专家还报告了一些国家特定的发展情况，记录如下。

奥地利：虽然照料老人的雇员、家政人员和社工的需求在增长，对残疾人照料雇员的需求总体保持不变。不过，照料残疾人的高素质人才的就业前景还是很好的。

保加利亚：虽然没有数据，但有迹象显示，由于经济危机，在西班牙、希腊和意大利工作的保加利亚照料雇员正在回到保加利亚。这将暂时缓解保加利亚照料雇员的短缺。

丹麦：像很多其他国家一样，社区照料和家庭照料劳动力年龄相对偏大。另外，据报道，与许多其他职业相比，社会照料和健康照料助理职业具有较高的人员变动率。在丹麦农村地区，吸引和留住家庭照料雇员显得尤为困难。

法国：照料行业的雇主预计招聘困难的比例由 2011 年的 61%上升到 2012 年的 67%（2012 年所有行业的平均是 43%）。这些困难预计主要是缺少应征人员（77%），应征人员缺乏技术、文凭和积极性（67%），以及这一行业较差的工作环境（45%）。

德国：社区照料和家庭照料劳动力市场已经失衡。每 10000个空缺的职位，只有 3286 个注册的失业照料行业雇员具备合乎需要的培训。然而，不同地区的失业人员在照料行业找工作的数量差别很大。目前，劳动力市场苦于缺少有技能的雇员。

荷兰：由于荷兰政府降低成本的政策，福利工作的劳动力出现过剩情况，然而健康照料劳动力还是紧缺。

波兰：护士仍然移居到其他欧盟国家（尤其是北欧），那里的劳动待遇和工作环境更好。这加剧了波兰照料行业劳动力的紧缺。

葡萄牙：总体来看，目前葡萄牙不缺乏照料雇员，主要是高失业率造成的。这尤其适用于这一行业的高素质人群。目前，有超过十万的失业人员具有较高的学历，他们中的很多人在相关社会行业工作。然而，在一些地区，无资质或低资质的人员出现短缺。

西班牙：黑市经济看来是西班牙社区照料和家庭照料行业的一个问题。在这个不合法的劳动力市场，主要是低素质的妇女，尤其是移民，很活跃，劳动待遇和工作环境都不好。非法劳动力市场在危机时期增长了，因为非专业的照料更便宜。这是照料行业职业化和改善弱势群体雇员劳动待遇和工作环境的主要障碍。

英国：以往，英国的社会工作和社会照料具有以下特点：劳动力短缺，依赖加班、临时或经验不足的职员，管理差，官僚作风严重，缺少灵活的工作安排，需要在非社会工作时间工作，并且工作压力大，要求高。另外，这一行业的许多雇主雇佣欧盟和非欧盟国家的移民人员。

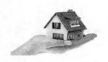

（三）发展预期

目前，经济危机使照料行业的劳动力紧缺得以缓解，在这一行业工作变得更受欢迎。长远来看，预计家庭照料雇员的紧缺会加剧，尤其是高素质的员工。照料人员的供应跟不上这一行业劳动力需求的增长。

各国专家提供的关于这个劳动力市场发展预期的信息记录如下。

奥地利：直到 2016 年，可以提供以下服务的社会照料专业人员的需求将每年增加 4500 人，或 3.4%，如，为老年人或残疾人提供照料同时也提供生活指导和社会咨询，需求增长的原因是人口年龄结构的变化。

到 2020 年，预计需要 6400 个额外的全职照料人员为老人、残疾人和其他依赖人群提供机动的服务。慢性病失能将导致这类人群更需要多年的照顾和照料而不是集中的药物治疗。

老人照料人员、家政人员和社工的需求在增长，残疾人照料护理人员的需求总体保持不变。

保加利亚：鉴于社区照料和家庭照料需求的增加，预计每年雇佣人员将增加 500 人至 1000 人。

丹麦：由于全球经济危机，劳动力市场短缺的整体问题比前几年减少很多。然而，从长远来看，老龄人口的增加和劳动力萎缩将导致家庭照料人员的短缺。

法国：家庭照料行业整体呈增长趋势。

荷兰：目前，社区健康照料的短缺相对较小（主要在资格水平3级，即中等职业水平，以及一些特殊专业），但未来几年这一短缺会加剧，尤其是高素质水平人员短缺。由于荷兰政府的降低成本政策，与福利相关的社会照料将出现劳动力过剩。雇主对家庭照料工人的任职资格、技术和技能的要求在提高，这主要是扩展协作的作用结果。

估计与健康相关的社会照料护士将短缺3000—5000名，有职业培训3级水平资格的工人将短缺几千名。

波兰：过去几年，健康行业长期照料机构的雇员数量有明显的下降，并且，预计未来几年这一下降会加剧。这主要是因为缺少新的和年轻的雇员，以及现有员工的退休。

欧洲经济政策研究所网络（ENEPRI）项目组对2031年照料相关专业员工数量发布了预测，这一预测对波兰尤其不利。预测指出，2011年有650000人在照料相关岗位工作，到2031年这些岗位只有350000人，大约是现在人数的一半。

葡萄牙：总体来看，由于高失业率，劳动力市场有资质和没有资质的雇员都没有明显的短缺。这一就业情况在中短期将持续。之后，将小幅度改善，因此，目前的劳动力市场过剩将持续相当长的一段时间。

2008—2011年，葡萄牙大约创造了120000个新的就业岗位，其中大约64000个是健康与社会照料工作。然而，与此同时，减少了480000个工作岗位。这些数字表明，今后健康与社会照料行业就业的增长估计每年最多为几千人。

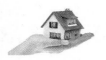

西班牙：为了确定2011—2015年新职位的数量，由西班牙工会组织，在个人自主和依赖照料系统框架下制订了两个不同的方案。一个理想的方案是，所有受益人都能得到专业的服务，这将创造261007个新职位，包括员工有食宿的照料、日间看护中心和家庭照料。

另一个限制性方案——25%的依赖人群可以得到财政补贴，由亲属来照料他们，其余75%由专业服务提供帮助——合计将创造195755个新的专业职位，由91202个有食宿的职位、45360个日间照料中心职位和59193个家庭照料服务组成。

英国：由于人口老龄化以及慢性病和残疾人数量的增加，预计英国社会照料服务的需求将迅速增加。估计从2010—2025年，英格兰成人社会照料工作数量将增加24%—82%。

三　照料与支持服务劳动力市场形势

外部因素影响残疾或有健康问题成年人的照料与支持服务劳动力市场的发展。这些因素为劳动力市场管理带来挑战，同时也提供解决方案。它们被确定为PESTLE分析规定的六个领域：政治领域、经济领域、社会领域、技术领域、法律领域和环境领域（见附录1）。

（一）政治和法律因素

不同国家关于残疾或有健康问题成年人照料与支持服务的

政治和法律政策框架差别很大。存在几方面的不同：照料政策总体目标；集权化和非集权化程度；提供正规照料人员的种类；直接支付系统对正规照料服务；资金结构。

1. 照料政策总体目标

尽管在欧洲不同国家中央政府对家庭照料的愿景设计千差万别，根据欧洲家庭照料报告，还是可以发现一些共同的特点（Genet 等，2012）。

一是各国政府对家庭照料愿景的设计通常是很笼统的，并且经常不定义关键概念或指明可测量的目标。

二是政府经常预见家庭照料的增长，常用来代替住家照料和医院照料。

三是家庭照料的构想通常涉及老龄化社会以及喜欢家庭照料的用户和他们的家人。家庭照料也要"适应社会的变化"（Genet 等，2012，p. 28）并符合提高生活质量的目标。关于这一方面，许多政府致力于提高残疾人的独立生活能力。

四是对非正规的照料人员与正规的家庭照料的支持似乎交织在一起，因为家庭照料被视为是促进非正规照料的途径。许多东欧国家，如保加利亚，甚至把家庭照料的构想纳入就业政策。一些国家用这个作为减少失业的手段，尤其是针对妇女，通过创造家庭照料的兼职工作解决就业问题。

五是一些政策文件把不同家庭照料服务类型之间更好地协作设为目标，如英国。

六是其他政策文件会涉及家庭照料相关的问题，包括照料

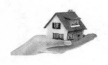

的质量水平与增加家庭照料劳动力（如在英国和荷兰）；增加民间社会在家庭照料中的作用（如荷兰和葡萄牙）；把家庭照料作为预防或确保社会隔离早期发现的手段。

除了这些概况，国家报告对一些国家特殊的发展政策进行了详细介绍。残疾或有健康问题成年人的照料与支持服务领域的主要发展总体方针归纳如下。

奥地利：奥地利长期照料的一个关键目标是帮助个人尽可能久地在家独立生活。这意味着社区照料服务今后将进一步扩大。另一个当务之急是在被照料人和照料人之间形成正式的合同协议，包括（经常未经申报）移民照料人。

保加利亚：随着立法改革的进行，在一贯的政策手段支持下，保加利亚从 2003 年开始进行社会服务权力下放的转型。人们普遍认同，由于人口老龄化以及老人和残疾人的家属对他们照料能力的下降，将导致社区照料服务需求的增长。这些服务将有助于提高残疾人的独立性，同时也改善他们家庭的生活质量。

丹麦：在丹麦，家庭照料服务被认为是干扰较少的照料形式。这样的照料被重新界定为提供给"健康消费者"而不是"病人"。这些新模式的实施发生在政府结构的去集权化趋势基础上，国家和地方董事会都变得更重要。公共管理的去集权化加速了丹麦政策去机构化的趋势。

法国：人口老龄化部分造成了照料需求的增长，法国照料系统的支出快速增加。降低成本政策提高了已经较高的家庭与社区照料水平。另一个鼓励社区照料的理由是激发病人的能力，使他们尽可能长久地独立生活。

德国：照料政策的目标是提高欧盟以外的国家移民人数。通过了一系列法律修正案来促进高技术人员和专家移民到德国。这将影响社区照料行业。欧盟以外有资质的照料人员现在更容易进入德国劳动力市场。

荷兰：荷兰内阁认为社区健康与社会照料是当务之急。作为组成部分的社区量身定制的照料为市民提供了更好的服务，并且更早发现问题。为此，新内阁延续了提高社区照料水平的政策并将职责转移到社区水平。与此同时，通过关注疾病与残疾的预防、自我管理与非正规照料等措施，重点降低专业照料的需求，与过去相比，客户和他们的亲属负责安排照料。

波兰：目前，波兰关于长期照料没有系统的方法。然而，法律调整已经为改善情况做了准备。这包括引入代金券计划，用代金券的家庭可以为家庭成员购买所需照料产品或服务，以及在健康保障行业强制性缴纳照料保险。

葡萄牙：在葡萄牙，现行的公共预算、债务合并过程以及其他降低国家在经济运营上的作用的措施都强有力地影响着国家政策。卫生、教育和社会照料服务正在进行合理化改革，国家作为市场监管人的作用在加强。三五年后，这些措施将使国家福利职责从公共资源获得的资金减少。这将增加私人照料提供者的压力，他们要支持需要的人群，保持适当的质量标准以及属地覆盖。

西班牙：鉴于目前的经济和财政危机，西班牙政府推行了几项措施，对于维持和创造照料劳动力市场高质量工作职位发

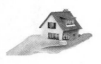

挥了间接作用。最重要的一个变化是2012年2月通过了劳动力改革政策。政府坚信它的措施有助于维持就业水平，一旦经济开始好转就能看见显著的效果。另外，"西班牙就业计划2012—2014"强调了促进新兴经济活动就业的重要性，例如，正在增长的社会与卫生行业，尤其是与服务相关的活动。

英国：在英国，有几条相关法规有利于发展社区照料。残疾人在公共生活的各个领域享有平等的权利，这会促进各行各业和劳动力市场发展，影响社会照料提供者，使社区照料的独立性、保障和质量得到改善。同时，推行了直接付费和个人照料预算，使得使用服务的人对个人照料需求有更多的选择和掌控。政府谋求削减居住照料的费用，将这些资金投资到社区照料服务，从而提高直接付费和个人预算的使用。

2. 集权化程度

正规照料领域制定政策和执行任务的集权化程度（国家对地区或地方政府）各不相同。欧洲家庭照料报告显示，许多国家制定家庭照料政策的职责适度分散。家庭健康照料的政策制定比社会家庭照料更集中。政府控制最集中的国家是比利时、塞浦路斯、法国和瑞士，而最分散的是冰岛和意大利（Genet等，2012）。一些国家正在研究这些计划，例如，奥地利、保加利亚、丹麦和荷兰，这些国家的记者报道了正规照料领域政策制定的增加，以及任务向下级机关执行出现分散的情况有所增加。

国家研究分析显示，人们享受社区照料或机构照料的资格条件，以及照料评估过程都因国家以及照料类型的不同而异。在大多数国家的研究里，公共财政资助的社区照料服务都有正式的合格标准（除了保加利亚社区照料的部分类型）。

照料的评估大多是由地方政府和组织负责。只有荷兰，国家照料评估中心在政府指导方针的框架内决定个人照料和家庭照料的确切的合格标准。

3. 正规照料的供应商

正规照料的供应商因国家而异，并且涵盖许多不同的组织，包括公立机构、私人公司、第三方组织以及非政府组织（如教堂和宗教组织）。通常，照料供应商是不同类型的混合。葡萄牙的情况说明了供应商种类的多样性。

葡萄牙的社区照料

仁慈的上帝屋：这些组织已经存在几个世纪了。传统的仁慈屋为穷人提供基本的健康援助，随着时间的推移，它们的活动变得多样化——帮助儿童、老人和残疾人，提供专业培训以及与社会排斥和失业做斗争。尽管是天主教会授权的，葡萄牙的仁慈屋不受教会高层的管理。

教区中心和其他宗教组织：正如宗教秩序规定的，教区中心由辖区主教在他管理的教区建立。教区中心提供的服务范围因中心的大小、城市化程度和其他社区因素而不同，包括为老人提供住所，业余时间和日间照料中心，家庭和临时照料服务，学前和幼儿园中心，音乐学校和其他文化、教育、体育、休闲、社会和健康照料活动。

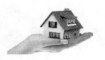

互惠或互利协会：起源于中世纪的兄弟会，它们的第一个现代形式是 1840 年创造的相互信用机构。互利会是为会员提供服务的组织，尤其是对社会保障领域的补充，如健康保险、疾病与退休金、补贴的卫生服务与药店，日间照料中心与学前和幼儿园中心。它们也提供优惠的贷款、诉讼援助、奖学金、假日中心和其他服务。

合作社：开始于 19 世纪，1974 年军事政变后得到显著发展。一些合作社提供社会与健康照料服务。

其他非营利机构：包括社会团结基金会和积极提供社会与健康服务的社会活动志愿者协会。

商业组织：包括保险公司、基金管理公司、为老年人和残疾人提供照顾与居住照料的公司。

其他供应商：与正规照料组织一样，个人和家庭也可以注册成为社会照料服务供应商。他们服从于适用于组织供应商的相似管理条例，并享受与组织供应商相同的鼓励措施。这一范畴包括三种服务：儿童照料人员、家政人员、老人与残疾人寄养家庭。

有些国家的照料供应商种类相当少。例如，在丹麦、荷兰和英国，社区服务主要由公立机构和私人公司提供。这个报告里研究的一些国家，如保加利亚、波兰、葡萄牙和荷兰，记者报道了照料服务外包给私人供应商的情况在增加。

4. 直接付费系统

在所有研究的国家里，照料和支持服务都是由国家提供。也有一些国家，直接付费系统与正规服务并存。直接付费系统给客户一个个人预算，他们可以自己购买专业照料或者付钱给家庭成员让他们来照料。某种意义上，客户成了雇主。

在欧洲各地，直接付费的定义与执行在许多方面有所不同（Genet 等，2012）：（1）补贴规则，受益人的数量和类型；（2）目标人群，客户或者非正规照料提供人；（3）资金（与实物福利相比）以及与他们相关的社会权利；（4）对资格的考察过程和预算的特殊使用，以及对提供的服务质量的评估；（5）只有现金福利或有现金和实物福利两种选择。

直接付费系统与提供照料服务并存的国家为奥地利、保加利亚、西班牙、英国和荷兰。

5. 资金结构

欧洲国家照料和支持服务最常见的资金来源为：（1）税收（国家、地区或市政征收的）；（2）保险（各种形式的强制或自愿的）；（3）捐款和第三方出资（照料可以由慈善组织提供，私人捐助的非政府组织或会员费，有些国家从欧盟获得资金）；（4）自掏腰包（通过税收或社会保险支付的照料要求客户共同负担）。

通常，资金是这些来源的混合。只有在丹麦，税收是资金的唯一来源（Genet 等，2012）。

在深入研究多数国家中发现，基于税收的公共供给以法律形式存在，国家保险提供津贴给长期医疗保健与社会照料。一些案例显示，人们必须自己承担一部分照料费用。

这 10 个国家的资金结构总结如下。

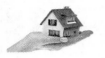

奥地利：相关的津贴收入和实物福利混合。

保加利亚：社会服务资金基于一个公共资金的再分配系统，以集中和分散的方式进行分配。社会服务的主要资金来源是国家预算和人力资源发展运营项目（一个欧洲社会基金项目）。

丹麦：医疗保健系统的资金由税收负担，这意味着大多数服务是免费的，主要参与者，包括购买人和大多数提供者，是公共的。法律允许地方政府在家政和其他一些与健康不相关的支出方面设定费用的有限自由。

法国：资金来源由税收和客户共同负担。

德国：德国为照料实施了一个公共保险系统，基于的原则是保险系统成员目前的交费直接用于资助寻求照料人员的支出。不同于资本存量系统，个人缴费被储蓄并积累，账单到期即付的资助系统用等量的收益来资助新的支出。因此赤字部分必须通过提高国债或改变交费水平来解决。

荷兰：荷兰照料系统的资金部分基于税收，根据特殊医疗支出法案（AWBZ）和社会支持法案（WMO），部分基于保险。基本健康保险法案包括了家庭医生、医院和药房的费用。其他费用人们可以通过补充医疗保险来支付。残疾人社区照料主要由 AWBZ 和 WMO 资助。通常，人们也必须自己支付照料费用的一部分。除了公共照料，荷兰也有私人照料。

波兰：在波兰，社区照料有两个主要资金来源：公共资金，部分基于保险，部分基于税收；私人费用，支付给提供长期照料的公司。

葡萄牙：除了商品和服务销售、财产性收入、私人转让（包括捐款和遗产）以及其他各种收入来源，这个行业很大一部分收入来源于政府转让和其他公共捐款与补助。

西班牙：一般而言，公共机构负责确定市民的权利和决定提供什么样的服务，以及分配资金。实际的服务供应由公立和私立代理商分担。西班牙总体社会服务系统分为三级行政管理：国家、地区和地方。使用服务的人也承担部分费用，这取决于他们的具体情况。

英国：英国社区照料的大部分资金来自于中央政府的税收支持拨款。政府也给地方机构特殊的拨款，但很大一部分支出来源于地方政府自己的资金，主要是征收的居住税。除了通过从事商业活动创造收入，地方政府也希望实现社会服务预算的节约。

随着照料需求和照料费用的增长，通常客户自己必须负担很大的份额。例如，在荷兰和德国都是这样。

特殊劳动力市场资金结构的管理措施因国家而异。国家之间有很大的预算差异。一些国家，如保加利亚，更多地依赖欧盟资金如欧洲社会基金项目，而北部成员国更多地依赖国家资金。

（二）经济因素

照料行业是一个重要的经济行业和主要的工作来源。目前，本研究里所有的国家都受经济危机的影响，一些国家比另

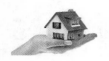

一些国家遭受经济危机更严重。经济危机对社区照料劳动力市场的影响方式不同。多数国家健康与社会照料行业面临着削减成本的问题。某种程度上，降低成本限制了这一行业的劳动力需求。例如在荷兰，由于大量减少社会照料，社会照料人员的需求也减少了。在英国，社工和地方政府雇佣的照料人员面临着报酬减少和报酬冻结。受地方政府委托的私营照料服务供应商也受到了影响。

在不繁荣的时期，社区照料比机构照料更为重要的金融观点将导致更多的社区照料需求，同时减少机构照料需求。

从需方来看，经济危机使得公共照料行业的工作比私人行业更有吸引力，私人行业危机的影响通常更深远。这意味着更多的社区照料劳动力需求。例如在保加利亚，在劳动力市场日益恶化的情况下，社会照料服务对失业者来说更有吸引力，它的总失业率是12%，而年轻人的失业率是27%，50岁以上人的失业率是45%。

降低失业率，尤其是年轻人的失业率，是经济危机中的重要议程，劳动力市场措施被更广泛地运用。在这种环境下，社区照料的劳动力可能会更多。例如，荷兰内阁近来为2013年和2014年额外拨出了5000万欧元，专门解决年轻人的失业问题。一半的钱用于"学校激励器"项目，鼓励中级职业水平的学生继续学业，尤其是在劳动力短缺的领域，如健康照料。另一半政府资金分配给市政当局组织的地方计划和荷兰就业服务，帮助年轻人找到工作。此外，还将任命一名青年就业大使。

（三）社会因素

1. 社会人口因素

最重要的影响社区照料劳动力市场的社会人口因素是快速的人口老龄化。预计，欧盟 27 国加上挪威和瑞士，老年人（65 岁及以上）的数量将从 2010 年的八千九百万增加到 2030 年的一亿两千五百万（Rodrigues 等，2012）。

图 3 比较了欧盟 27 国以及 10 个研究国老年依赖比例的预计发展情况。这个指标是经济上不活跃的老人（65 岁及以上）的数量和工作年龄人群数量（15 到 64 岁）的比值。

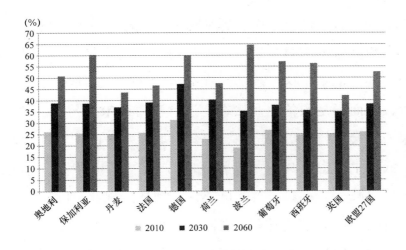

图 3　欧盟 27 国和 10 个研究国老年依赖比例预测

来源：欧盟统计局。

总的来说，预计欧盟 27 国老年依赖比例将从 2010 年的

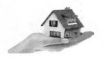

25.9% 提高到 2030 年的 38.3% 和 2060 年的 52.6%。这一增长趋势也适用于这里研究的 10 个国家，尽管增长的速度有所不同。

2010 年，这一比例最高的是德国、葡萄牙和奥地利（分别是 31.2%、26.7% 和 26.1%），最低的是波兰、荷兰和西班牙（19.0%、22.8% 和 24.7%）。2060 年，预计这一比例最高的是波兰、保加利亚和德国（分别是 64.1%、60.3% 和 59.9%），最低的是英国、丹麦和法国（42.7%、43.5% 和 46.7%）。

由于长寿老人的增加以及患有痴呆、慢性病和残疾人数量的增加，照料人员需求增加。与此同时，人口老龄化也导致劳动力供应的减少。

其他影响社区照料劳动力市场的社会人口因素是年轻人数量的下降，这是低出生率和新型家庭模式的出现造成的。

作为低出生率的结果，进入职业培训的年轻人将减少。荷兰国家报告记录了这一趋势，在荷兰，年轻人更愿意进入预备高等教育而不是预备职业培训。这意味着，未来荷兰高素质的健康与社会照料人员将增加，但具有职业水平的护士将紧缺。

低出生率也将减少可以照顾自己老年亲属的年轻一代的人数。这将减少非正规照料的可能性，增加正规照料的需求。

另一个社会人口因素，在西班牙的报道中很明确，是新家庭模式的出现，例如，单身家庭数量的增加，以及女性更加普遍地进入劳动力市场。这意味着提供非正规照料的女性将减少，正规照料的需求将增加。

2. 社会文化因素

社会文化因素影响残疾或有健康问题成人照料与支持服务的劳动力市场。这方面一个重要因素是正规照料对非正规照料的比例。欧洲家庭照料报告显示，在欧盟大多数国家，非正规照料提供者，如家人、邻居和朋友提供了平均大约60%的家庭照料个人需求（Genet 等，2012）。在希腊和一些中欧国家，90%的家庭照料由家人提供。相反，在丹麦只有15%的家庭照料由家庭成员提供。

图4提供了涉及照料行业劳动强度的照料正规化程度详细信息。图的左边显示了照料行业劳动力相对于65岁及以上总

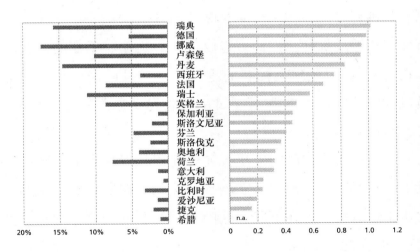

图4　照料行业正式雇佣的人相对于65岁及以上人口的百分比（左）以及照料行业正式雇佣的人相对于用户的比例（右）

注：法国的数据涉及2003年和2008年。

来源：Rodrigues 等，2012。

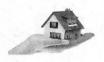

人口的百分比。右边显示了照料行业劳动力相对于 65 岁及以上正规照料服务用户的比例。后一个指标也可以看作照料质量的替代投入指标。较高的分数意味着较高的劳动强度正规化水平。

从图 4 可以得出以下结论。

首先，图的左边显示了照料配置的正规化程度，反映了长期照料劳动力对老年人口的相对重要性。挪威、丹麦和瑞典是去家庭化的典型，这些国家福利需求的满意度高，并独立于家庭，是国家的责任，尽管后者近来又转回为更多的家庭责任。

其次，图的右边显示了劳动力与照料服务老年用户的比例。某种程度上，体现了照料服务与开支的关系，就像前面章节详细描述的那样。然而，造成差异的是兼职工作的流行（例如在荷兰），以及现金福利的重要性，它可以用来支付家庭成员或移民照料员工的费用（如在奥地利或意大利）（Rodrigues 等，2012）。

在一些被研究的国家里，如奥地利和保加利亚，可以看到近来家庭照料中正规照料在增加。例如，在奥地利，家庭成员的非正规照料程度在下降。这归功于社会的变化，即工作女性的数量在增加，而且估计会进一步增加。对于支持和平衡工作与家庭生活，专业照顾和照料服务变得更加重要。

在保加利亚或多或少可以看到相同的发展，那里对家庭和家人深度依赖是惯例。然而，社会的变化使得一个人献身于家庭变得困难，尤其是当家庭成员有重病需要照顾的情况下。如果人们不得不照顾患病的亲属，他们必须放弃工作，这将降低整个家庭的生活质量。尽管机构长期照料与保加利亚的传统完全相悖，但也成为可行的办法。国家从财政上支持需要家庭照料的人，他们有家庭和亲属，国家付钱给他们的亲属去照顾他们，这是合理和有效的。

然而，在其他国家，如荷兰，政策开始向更多的非正规照料转移，强调减少专业照料需求，例如通过促进疾病与残疾预防，自我管理与非正规照料来实现。客户的亲属承担了更多的照料责任。

非正规照料的缺点是照料残疾亲属的人完全或部分地远离了劳动力市场。

3. 社会经济因素

第三个相关的范畴是社会经济因素。正如已提到的，经济危机严重影响了市民的健康与福利。一些国家恶劣的经济形势会导致卫生与社会问题的增加，从而使得对照料人员的需求增加。

（四）技术因素

技术为健康与社会照料行业带来了重大发展。

医学知识和治疗方法的发展使得平均寿命延长，这将导致今后长期照料需求的增加。高龄也导致得严重疾病的可能性增加。因此，不仅总的照料人员的需求在增加，高素质照料人员的需求预计也将增加。

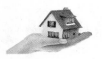

社区照料的劳动生产率提高了，尽管利润相对较低。理论上，生活辅助技术运用的增加，例如家庭自动化、远程监护和数字化服务，以及材料的创新应用于个人照料等，导致了社区照料具有更有效和更高的劳动生产率，从而减少需求。最近由未来技术研究所执行的 CARICI（"照料与信息通信技术"的缩写）研究计划显示，在欧洲有许多不同类型的信息通信技术支持照料行业的例子，它们是成功、便宜和有用的范例（Carretero 等，2013）。然而，照料行业将维持劳动力相对密集的状况。荷兰的经验表明，技术创新对照料质量的影响大于对照料人员劳动生产率的影响。

客户对生活辅助技术越来越多的运用将对家庭照料劳动力产生影响。新技术的发展将帮助人们使用这些技术。例如，在英国，担任各种各样社区角色的社会照料工作人员需要掌握生活辅助技术，"照料技能"向家庭照料劳动力提供了与生活辅助技术相关的综合技能、知识、理解与实践的指导，生活辅助技术的发展还为英国引入了一类新型的家庭照料人员，即辅助技术支持人员。

（五）环境因素

最后一个领域是环境。然而，这个因素对照料劳动力市场的影响是微不足道的。10 个被研究的国家大多如此。只有在葡萄牙，环境部门不断地为开发社会的和有意义的工作提供机会，以帮助失业的人更好地为残疾人服务。

四　劳动力供应

虽然对照料供应者的需求在增长，由于劳动力老龄化，工作人员的供应在下降。在丹麦、法国、荷兰、西班牙和英国，大约三分之一的照料人员的年龄大于 45 岁（Korczyk，2004；Ewijk 等，2002）。欧盟委员会统计，2000—2009 年，50 岁以上卫生与社会照料人员的数量增加了 20%（2012d）。到 2020年，人员更替的需要将导致七百万个职位空缺（还有一百四十万个新职位）（见 Korczyk，2004；Ewijk 等，2002；欧盟委员会，2012a）。委员会预测，到 2020 年，劳动力供求的不匹配将导致两百万健康照料人员短缺，其中一百万是长期照料供应者。因此，预计到 2020 年，欧洲健康照料人员将比需要的少 8.5%。

五　雇员特征

有关雇员特征，上面的调查和报告已经强调了健康劳动力的几个特点。首先，欧盟 27 国健康与社会照料劳动力组成主要是女性。其次，与总劳动力相比，健康与社会照料劳动力的教育程度相对较高，至少在欧盟 15 国是这样。如果包括新成员国，这一行业具有高等职业或大学教育的雇员百分比就下降到整体经济行业的平均水平。

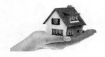

　　这一行业雇员的高教育水平也反映在劳动力的预测上。2010—2020 年预计将产生 800 万个健康照料工作，大多数将给高学历的人（500 万左右），然后是中等学历水平的人（300 万左右），只有约 20 万个工作给低水平资历的人。

　　健康与社会照料行业兼职工人的比例也比整体经济行业高很多，为 31.6%，而经济行业整体平均比例为 18.8%。一个值得注意的特点是健康与社会照料员工相对较低的报酬。欧盟委员会指出，尽管技术水平相对较高，工作环境通常要求很高，这个行业的整体小时工资比欧盟 27 国整体劳动力的平均小时工资要低。近几年，这一趋势变得更明显，这与该行业较高的女性雇员比例以及男女收入不平等有关。

第三章　招聘和保留措施

本章讨论了有关深入研究的 30 个招聘和保留雇员措施的分析结果。根据他们所支持的劳动力市场策略，本章解释了这些措施的分类情况，并简要介绍这一领域里国家层面的政策和行动。30 个招聘和保留雇员措施的要素概况如下。[①]

一　招聘和留用措施的类型

通过区分刺激劳动力供给与缓和劳动力需求的措施，可以将解决该领域劳动力短缺的对策分类。使用解决方案模型（见附录 1）作为起始点，确立了以社区为基础，招聘和保留雇员的残疾人照料的四个劳动力市场策略。

[①]　30 个案例的选择标准在介绍中有阐述。国家报告的附录对所研究的案例有详细的描述。

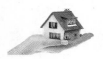

（1）针对劳动力储备来吸引新员工进入该行业。除了招聘的失业人员和目前不在社区照料中工作的其他团体，可能还包括现有移民群体和劳务移民。

（2）提升和促进潜在雇员的教育水平，比如，创造新型且具体的学习路径，或者通过一些活动来鼓励大家选择该行业公共机构组织的教育培训。

（3）改善现有员工的现状，充分发挥他们的潜能，同时劝阻他们不要离开该行业。可引入培训和再培训项目，让该行业更加专业化并且为现有员工提供更多的职业前景。

（4）提高本行业运作管理和劳动生产效率。这是通过让组织机构更有效地工作并提高员工生产力来减轻劳动力市场差异的一种方式，例如，使用新的技术和处理方法以及改善组织机构的功能职责。劳动密集型社区照料工作很难提高效率，但是革新的方法会对其产生积极的影响。

二　国家政策和行动

国家分析报告显示大多数国家对上述策略都有过尝试。然而，侧重点却各不相同。在一些国家如波兰，更侧重于改善社会保障的整体质量，继而提高照料工作的吸引力。丹麦和芬兰则着重提高这一行业的声誉。在一些像荷兰那样整体情况已经很好的国家，侧重点则是针对新的劳动力储备以及提高生产力。英国则引导人们进入该行业较低端的领域。这些措施的特殊性和差异性也很大，例如，在葡萄牙，虽然照料工作往往是重中之重，但是大多数劳动力市场目标是很宽泛的，相反在西班牙就会更狭小些，主要集中在家庭照料的工作上。

国家分析报告也揭示了各国之间有趣的相似之处。许多国家已经开发了远程监护项目（荷兰，西班牙和英国），增加了移民照料人员的数量（奥地利和丹麦），改变了照料组织结构（保加利亚，荷兰和西班牙），并引入了新的直接支付系统（奥地利，保加利亚，荷兰，西班牙和英国）。

三 案例研究：招聘和保留雇员的良策

本节概述了深入研究的 30 个招聘和保留雇员措施的主要内容。为了此项研究，这些案例依据它们阐述的最重要的策略进行了分类（有些案例涉及多个策略）。

策略 1：以劳动力储备为目标

这一策略主要是从劳动力储备，特别是失业人员中招聘家庭照护人员。这一举措主要结合了职业定位、资格预审、资格证明、工作经验、调节和后续支持以及劳动成本补贴。

社会工作和医护人员劳动基金会（奥地利）：这个举措针对对健康、护理或者社会工作感兴趣的维也纳失业人员。它会通过训练，帮助失业人员找到工作。根据个人适应性和语言能力等标准，求职者会通过一系列选拔程序，继而在完成培训后

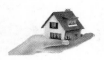

任职。协助组织即维也纳就业促进基金会会预先选择申请者。

移民照料（奥地利）：移民照料计划旨在帮助不以德语为母语的人成为合格的健康和社会照料工作者。在这一举措的框架内，感兴趣的移民可以通过个人咨询了解以社区为基础的照料就业情况。他们可以参加侧重德语语言技能的资格预选培训来帮助他们进入卫生和社会护理领域的职业培训。

残疾人助理（保加利亚）：此项国家计划的双重目标是为失业者提供工作机会以及为需要的人提供社区照料。该计划资助两种照料工作。个人助理职位是为了缓解需要时刻照料的残疾人的家庭压力，而社会救助任务则是为了帮助严重患病的残疾人及孤寡老人，这包括管理他们的闲暇时间，帮助他们融入社会。残疾人亲属可以申请个人助理职位。

工作轮岗（丹麦）：工作轮岗计划旨在改善现有员工的专业发展，同时，为失业人员或新晋的合格员工提供以社区为中心的照料工作。目前，正在接受培训的员工的职位会为失业人员或新晋员工开放，这些职位暂时由失业人员填补。因此，这一举措不仅帮助失业人员丰富工作经验（策略1），而且为现有员工提升资质（策略3，如后文所述）。

2012年激励计划（葡萄牙）：2012年激励计划旨在帮助已经注册失业超过六个月的求职者提供寻求就业和技能提升的财政支持。此项计划补贴受雇人员连续六个月工资的50%。除此之外对特殊的求职者会有10%的额外补贴，包括残疾人求职者。申请补贴的雇主在计划结束后要提供永久劳动合同或者至少可以续期六个月的定期劳动合同。

EIP 计划（葡萄牙）：EIP 计划为求职者提供 12 个月的社会服务类临时工作；它针对处境困难的群体，特别是长期失业人士。此项计划的主要目的是通过帮助维持或提高求职者的个人能力和专业技巧，让他们与劳动力市场接轨，减少求职者与市场的隔离和消极丧志感，从而提高求职者未来的就业能力。

单程票计划（英国）：在曼彻斯特运作的单程票计划（STP）旨在帮助失业人员和弱势群体获得有关社会保障的知识、技能和工作经验。选择的主要标准则是参与者想从事健康与社会照料工作的决心和意愿，而非之前是否有在这一行业的工作经验或学历。STP 的职业培训方法是通过一个综合性计划（"单程票"）来帮助工作者获得多种职业选择的核心技能和经验。此项目的则是为劳动力人口创造灵活性。该计划包括 4 周的入职培训、5 次工作实习、每次工作实习大约 12 周左右，由健康与社会照料供应商提供。这些工作可能会涉及成人护理、儿童照料、心理健康领域，参与者会在综合医院或者与患有学习障碍症的人一起工作，完成该计划的参与者会有比较坚实的基础用来申请该行业的长期工作。

策略 2：提升和促进教育

这一策略旨在招募能够从事社会照料学生，并帮助他们留在该行业。策略目的是为愿意并能够留在社区照料行业的工作者提供机会。这一策略的范例可以分成三组：活动和教育指

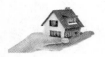

导，社会照料的学徒制以及导师制。

活动和教育指导

男孩节（奥地利）：在一年一度的男孩节，男孩们开始知道展示男性角色的照料护理和教育职业。男孩节的长期目标是：①让更多男性进入典型女性主导的职业；②打破社会固有的观念；③改善社会工作和健康护理的职业形象；④帮助男孩成长为阳光积极的男性。

此外，有许多面向十二岁及以上男孩的职前指导的讲座在一年中成功举办。这些讲座为男孩们展示了有关社会照护工作和社会文化的电影视频。此项计划也有自己的网站。

展望未来计划（德国）：展望未来计划在2010—2011年进行，旨在通过向中学生提供信息并且鼓励青少年考虑照料行业从而解决该行业劳动技能短缺的问题。开发人们如何在健康照料行业建立社交网络的手册，并由该社交网络成员传授训练课程框架。同时，展望未来计划也引入一种同伴学习的培训方法，让护理学校的学员为中学生讲课。这种方法与在护理照料机构的两周实习相结合，实习学生会由现任高级职员指导。

学徒制

邻里培训公司（荷兰）：邻里培训公司是一个社区健康卫生培训和社会照料的新概念。它旨在帮助参与者得到与自己居住区医疗保健和福利事业直接相关的工作经验。邻里培训公司能够完成居民自己无能为力而市政当局不能给予他们帮助的散活。

INOV-SOCIAL（葡萄牙）：INOV-SOCIAL 会向高等职业教育应届毕业生提供通常为期九个月的社会照料领域的专业学徒制培训。这一举措的主要目标是提高毕业生的专业技能，并且促进他们融入社会照料体系内的劳动市场，继而改善所提供的服务质量。

导师制

针对外国留学生的就业指导系统（丹麦）：该系统为非丹麦裔学生提供有关健康或社会照料领域的就业指导，鼓励他们完成学业，减少辍学率，并且为社区照料领域的职业做更好的准备。在该系统中，每个学生都会配有一名导师。导师会由健康保障或社会照料行业的老师或志愿者担任，他们都是依然在该行业工作或已经退休的人员。导师制系统由安排工作实习的网络帮助协调，并且担任导师与学生的中间联系人。

策略3：改善现有员工现状

第三个策略是通过改善现有员工职业资格或者为他们提供其他职业发展的手段来预防现有员工离职。虽然这是主要目标，但是升级社区照料行业也会对潜在雇员更有吸引力，并有助于招聘雇员。该战略采取的措施包括：对该行业进行专业化升级；提供培训和继续教育项目来提高员工的专业知识、技能和学习动力。与此同时，为员工提供更多的职业前景，并采取更加新型现代的培训和教育方法，如在线学习和工作经验的专业认证等。

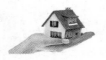

行业专业化

照料行业职员发展专业化（德国）：行业专业化从2009—2012年开始运行，旨在发展照料行业劳动力管理技能，比如，人力资源开发领域，参与者有机会了解更多职业课程并且获得尽可能多的以实践为核心的相关知识。这些课程将理论管理与工作实践相结合。行业专业化旨在培养以社区照料为基础的服务对系统化和策略化的人力资源发展的需求意识。护理学院的人力资源顾问会帮助解答有关社区照料服务涉及人力资源相关的问题，并且协助人力资源开发系统的设计。

社会工作者的新职业角色（波兰）：该项目开发了一个新的社会工作标准，被称为"社区组织模式"，它描绘了社会工作者如何支持受到贫困、边缘化或社交排外威胁的个体，并通过与他们直接合作的方式来帮助这些个体重新融入社区和就业。与此相匹配的标准是对于能直接联系客户和能按照准则工作的社会工作者给予财务奖励。2013—2014年，全国约有3000名社会工作者接受了为期两天的新标准培训。

社会照料人力发展计划（SCWDP）（英国）：该计划是一项区域性举措，通过向威尔士的地方当局提供资助的方式来为其他地区开展SCWDP合作。这些合作伙伴负责在该地区公有和私营的社会照料劳动力的SCWDP培训资助的发展、规划、监督和测评。他们也会通过向管理人员提供招聘和保留雇员相关事宜的培训，来制订社会照料服务提供者的招聘和保留雇员措施。最终目的是增加有资质、技能和知识的雇员比例，从而提高该地区社会服务的质量和管理水平。

员工培训

社会助理和家庭助理服务（保加利亚）：保加利亚在2007—2012 年提供过资金来支持那些帮助不能自理的残疾人的社会助理和家庭助理人员，让他们的技能和工作动力得以提高。这三个阶段方案主要旨在提高在社会工作领域有经验的下岗或在职人员的技能。此方案的总目标是加强和改善社会助理服务，并以社区为基础的社会服务形式来发展家庭助理服务，帮助经常被社会排斥或不能依靠护理机构的人群。该方案的具体目标则是为社会服务行业创造新的就业机会，以为相关人员寻求更多工作，以及提高所有社会助理和家庭助理的劳动技能和工作动力。

慢性病继续教育（丹麦）：在许多欧洲国家，为了控制慢性病发病率的上升趋势，社区照料领域专业人员的技能需要得到提升。这项丹麦倡议旨在加强卫生领域专业人员在综合实践、社区照料和医院的职业发展。这项倡议包括与临床实践密切联系的一系列课程和培训模块，其目的是提高现有劳动力的能力，来控制社区照料领域中的慢性病。该计划的前提是，以团队为基础，并以个人为中心，满足个人需求而量身定做的慢性病控制方法，在该基础上提供技能开发。

资质作为提高照料服务质量的关键（波兰）：大波兰地区的这个项目集中在对已经积极参加长期照料工作的人员进行培训，其中大部分人是正式员工。该项目以讲座和实践相结合的

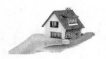

形式培训，涵盖了有健康问题的老年人和残疾人的照料方法等主题。

员工教育的新方法

社区照料工作经验的专业认证（法国）：基于经验的法国专业认证体系（Validation des Acquis de l'Expérience，VAE），认证考试可以使至少具有三年工作经验的个人获得专业资格证书或文凭。VAE对那些可以证明自己有工资、自主创业或做志愿工作的人开放。报考者必须登记相关的工作经验，回答有关资格的问题并进行口头考试。认证程序由多个部门组织，每个部门负责确定候选人完全满足在其行业中VAE的各项要求。

照料行业的在线学习（eLiP）（德国）：在线学习计划旨在促进照料行业在线学习传播。通过提供中枢的在线基础设施，个人可以用合理的价格访问，而不是选择市场上现有的在线学习产品。eLiP项目经理认为，针对照料行业量身定做的软件解决方案可以在该行业得到接受和广泛使用。

专业证书（西班牙）：在西班牙专业验证体系里，每个专业证书由多个"技能单元"组成，通常为两个或者三个，每个技能单元都与短期培训模块直接相关。如若要得到最终的专业证书则需先完成所有技能单元的证明。专业证书的内容、技能单元、专业背景和专业档案正式由皇家法令规定，国家批准并颁布。劳动部和教育部是负责此过程的主要国家机构。自治社区及其劳动和教育当局负责执行区域级认可体系。

策略 4：提高管理和劳动生产率

职能、组织或应用技术的创新变化，以及这三个要素的组合可以改善社区照料行业的运营管理和劳动生产率。除了削减劳动力成本外，新的工作方式也可以使该行业对现有雇员和潜在员工更具吸引力，从而增加招聘和留住雇员的可能性。根据发生的变化，阐明这一策略的案例可以划分为四个小组：新职能；组织和指导照料工作的新方式；科技创新；为帮助残疾人更加积极地进入劳动力市场、教育和社会领域而提供的新型就业和交通服务。

新职能

可见链接（荷兰）：在 2009—2012 年，该计划促进了（特别是在社会经济和健康弱势的社区中）高效技能社区护士的成本效益部署。社区护士的职责是通过将公民与住宅、疾病预防和健康与社会照料领域的地方各个机构组织联系起来，继而解决他们，尤其是弱势群体的问题。除了协助医疗卫生和社会保障外，护士还会在人们的家中提供照料服务。可见链接的主要目的是改善社区照料的连贯性。

医护人员新职业（波兰）：该措施为新进入长期护理领域的医护人员提供职业培训。在护士的监督指导下，医护人员会完成一些原本由资深护士做的简单的护理工作。这个新职业已经被列入国家教育部保留的专业职业列表（波兰职业和专业分类），完成相关职业培训后，医护人员可以正式注册登记。

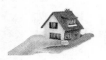

组织和指导照料工作的新方式

邻里照料（荷兰）：该项目提供小型、自主组织的高技能社区工作人员团队来全权负责护理照料在家的客户。这些团队可以通过志愿者的帮助或者协助客户提供正规的健康与社会照料系统的服务。必要时，他们会提供上门家庭护理照料。这些当地团队是被一个小但有能力的国家组织资助的。此项目的目的是提高家庭照料的质量和效率，使社区护士的工作更井然有序、更有吸引力。

独立生活（西班牙）：独立生活是吉普斯夸省的直接支付项目，旨在促进18岁以上居住在自己家中的残疾人的自主独立生活。受益人自主管理自己的照料预算，负责招聘其私人助理，无论是亲戚或是合格的专业人士。每个受益人平均有2—3名私人助理来为他们做他们自己无法完成的日常事情。残疾人自己监督这些支持，但是私人助理不负责决策。

SSI集团（西班牙）：SSI（整合社会服务）集团是一个毕尔巴鄂的非营利的专业社会照料合作社。SSI集团拥有集自治、管理自主化、参与平等化、财产集体化、交流合作、分散型人力资源结构为一体的合作模式。其主要价值观念则是个人成长、持续培训、专业标准维护、社会举措支持以及社会增值福利的再投资。SSI集团的目标之一则是帮助非正式的护理人员取得正式的专业资格，并在此过程中，增加他们工作的价值。

科技创新

诺福克辅助技术（英国）：该项目旨在发展一种专门从事

辅助技术社会工作者，即辅助技术支持人员（AT）。辅助技术支持人员会对（潜在）服务用户进行评估，例如，在辅助技术上的需求，无论是独立的设备还是远程监护设备。他们还负责转包设备的安装，并为各郡的不同群体提供培训、意识提升研讨会、讲座以及临床实习等。

为残疾成年人提供的新型就业和交通服务

社会创业（保加利亚）：2009—2011 年，社会创业补助资金计划旨在创造成功的社会企业新模式来改善现有企业。这样做的目的是创造稳定的工作，特别是在服务行业，因为弱势群体无法参与到正常的工作中去。此项计划促进和支持社会企业，强化意识并且促进在该领域中多方组织参与的相关合作。

工作建立和服务支持（ESATs）（法国）：由国家资助的ESATs 旨在为患有严重残疾并影响正常找工作的残疾人提供工作。通过帮助残疾人融入社会，ESAT 的医疗和社会工作者成为当地合作伙伴网络的一部分，并且可以为他们的客户提供住房信息、预防医学课程、照料甚至文化活动。因此，他们不仅为残疾人提供工作，而且鼓励他们在工作之余的生活中融入社会。

PMR 交通服务（法国）：格勒诺布尔市的 PMR 交通服务使用能够承载多达五辆轮椅的小型巴士，并且巴士中配有铺钢轨的底板来固定轮椅。PMR 照料司机可以到家门口接人，但并不帮助他们从家里出来和送进家里。如有需要，其他照料人员会在 PMR 服务前或后提供帮助。PMR 照料司机大多数为男性，

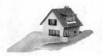

都是经过特殊培训的，他们要参加急救课程、平稳驾驶和预防驾驶课程、轮椅操控课程。他们定期接受残疾人士的专业培训，以便更好地了解各种残疾，并学习如何在旅途中对乘客负责。

第四章　结果、结论和影响

　　一般来说，有关招聘和保留照料人员措施的结果、结论和影响的信息是碎片化的。东欧国家尤其没有长期一贯的定期测评系统。其他欧洲国家的计划和项目也同样不会被经常评估。然而，通常情况下是由欧盟基金的受益组织，比如，欧洲社会基金进行义务测评。

　　此外，现有的许多计划仍在运作中，因此，只有部分计划可以被评估。还值得一提的是，一般来说，评估员工短缺的劳动力市场政策的有效影响并非易事。最近一份荷兰的可行性研究报告证实了医疗行业评估劳动力市场措施的困难。（Panteia等，2013）。研究表明，从短期来看，只有一些针对当前或预期的员工短缺的劳动力市场举措的影响可以得到适当评估。从长远看，更多的劳动力市场举措的影响部分可以更加充分地得到评估。然而，由于外部因素的影响总是会随着时间的推移而

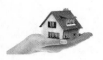

增加评估的难度，评估的可靠性将受到限制。现有数据的质量也必须得到提升，以便进行更准确的影响评估。即使如此，有些定量方面（例如，关于生产力的影响和劳动力市场措施的范围）和定性方面（比如劳动力市场发展的瓶颈和成功失败因素的识别）能够经常被评估。

一　案例研究：结果

所研究的 30 个案例大多数都是以定量或者定性的方式进行了监测或评估。总体上来讲，这些举措的结果和结论都是有前景的。但是，由于目标、战略、范围、区域规模和持续时间等方面的差异，难以比较所有举措的结果和影响。除此之外，用来衡量成功的指标也是不尽相同的。创造就业或总是提供有关就业机会的信息也不是所有举措的直接目标。有时候，也使用其他指标，例如，参与措施的人数，可用地点的数量，积极参与的人数和成功完成的人数。

报告的这一部分概述了 30 个案例研究的结果。这些举措的结论和影响简要论述如下。

策略 1 的结果：把储备劳动力作为目标

社会工作和医护人员劳动基金会（奥地利）：2003 年 1 月至 2007 年 9 月，740 名家庭护理帮助者、206 名护士助理和 20 名认证医护人员以及护士完成了职业培训；这组人群中的 95%

找到了工作。9—12 个月后,该组人群的就业率保持在 90% 左右。

移民照料(奥地利):大约有 350 人从 2012 年 7 月至 9 月到访了中心联络点。许多人都是通过一次短暂但内容丰富的交谈而得到帮助的。该中心大概举办了 200 次综合和个人咨询会,由于预算限制,2012 年仅举办了一次 18 人的资格预审课程。

残疾人助理(保加利亚):该计划在 2005—2011 年创造了 8 万多个就业机会。

工作轮岗(丹麦):2012 年,一些项目仍在进行中,估计有 770 人参加临时工作。在一批完成轮岗项目的 291 名临时工中,有 78% 的人在项目结束后两周内受雇。此外,另一批 286 名临时工中有 63% 在轮岗完成两周之后就业,而没有参加项目的比较组就业率则为 43%。现有员工对该行业的满意度的提升和成长机会的增多,表明该行业保留雇员是很成功的,尽管目前没有数据可以证实这点。

2012 年激励计划(葡萄牙):这一措施已经吸引了大量的受益组织:截至 2012 年 10 月,已有 3231 个组织和 5547 个工作岗位获得批准,487 个(15%)组织和 1006 个(18%)就业机会属于社会照料行业。此外,老人以及残疾人士照料服务新增职位 528 个,其中一半以上(52%)为社会工作者。

EIP 计划(葡萄牙):2011 年,这项措施涉及了 551038 名失业人员,其中 3478 人给老年人提供社会照料服务。2012 年

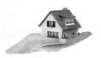

（截至 9 月），共涉及 44788 名失业人员，其中 3581 人向老年人提供社会照料服务。目前，社会照料服务在招标过程中的参与率呈上升趋势，这有可能是国家经济趋势下滑而导致的。

单程票计划（英国）：自 2009 年以来，约有 70 人参加了该计划。完成该计划后，约有 70% 的参与者进入卫生和社会照料领域就业。

策略 2 的结果：鼓励和促进教育

活动和教育指导

男孩节（奥地利）：2011 年，奥地利全国有超过 4000 名男孩参加了男孩节。来自 50 个学校的 1522 名男孩共参加了 111 个讲习班；来自 112 所学校的 2375 名男孩参观了教育和照料部门的 153 个机构；来自 26 所学校的 102 名男孩参与了 96 个机构的工作安置。

展望未来计划（德国）：没有可供使用的定量信息。

学徒制

邻里培训公司（荷兰）：邻里培训公司于 2011 年在多德雷赫特，哈勒姆，亨格洛，莱顿和乌得勒支市开展活动，每场活动有 15—22 个实习生职位。2010 年 1 月在海牙开展的项目中有约 100 个实习生职位。运营邻里培训公司项目的其他城市和地区还包括阿默斯特福，鹿特丹，维尼达尔和祖恩－肯恩梅兰。

INOV-SOCIAL（葡萄牙）：2010 年，有 1050 名人员参加此

项目，2011 年则为 1467 名。截至 2012 年 9 月，当该项目措施
被取代时，仍有 219 名人员从中受益。

导师制

针对外国留学生的就业指导系统（丹麦）：该项目从 2004
年的 15 对一对一的导师学生开始，到 2010 年，达到了 100 对。
目前该项目有 50 对。在接受调查的学生中，有 70% 表示他们
的导师为他们完成教育计划给予了重要支持；得到项目资助的
46% 的管理人员报告说，导师制令更多的移民青年成功完成学
业课程。

策略 3 的结果：改善当前员工现状
行业专业化

照料行业职员发展专业化（德国）：迄今为止，150 个社
区照料服务中的 180 人参加了其中一项课程。

社会工作者的新职业角色（波兰）：在初期阶段，共有 82
名社会工作者参加了此项目。2013—2014 年，约 300 名社会工
作者参加了宣传培训。

社会照料人力发展计划（SCWDP）（英国）：2010—2011
年，多达 127000 人参加了 SCWDP 资助的活动，比往年下降了
3.8 个百分比。期间获得资格的有 6500 人，比往年下降了 2.9
个百分比。在管理和社区照料培训领域获得的"指定资格"数
量略有下降（分别为 6% 和 4%）。但孩童照料资格增加
了 14%。

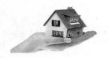

员工培训

社会助理和家庭助理服务（保加利亚）：在补助金计划的三个阶段框架内，共有 4152 名社会助理和 6785 名家庭助理就业。

慢性病继续教育（丹麦）：该项目的目标是在 2010—2012 年培训 3000 人；然而事实上有 5834 人参加了此项目。

资质作为提高照料服务质量的关键（波兰）：该项目吸引了 330 人参加。

员工教育的新方法

社区照料工作经验的专业认证（法国）：在 2011 年申请 VAE 的 51000 名候选人中，有近三分之一的人正在申请护理人员和家庭照料人员资格认证的职业培训。其中，6300 人申请了国家认可的护理辅助文凭；4800 人申请了国家认可的家庭照料助理文凭；还有 1900 人申请了作为家庭成员助理的家庭照料资格证书。

照料行业的在线学习（eLiP）（德国）：2008 年 eLip 的初始成员仅有七名。到 2012 年，该协会共有 20 名成员使用在线学习基础设施，并参加了 eLiP 提供的初级和高级研讨会。

专业证书（西班牙）：2012 年夏天，共有 787 人完成了家庭受扶养者的健康和社会照料服务的专业证书要求。刚进入初级评估阶段的人中只有 57% 获得了证书。在社会服务和社区服务部门中，有 1634 人获得了社会受扶养者的健康和社会照料专业证书，1202 人获得了家庭照料证书。在医疗从业中，有

352 人获得健康运输专业证书。

策略 4 的结果：提高经营管理和劳动生产率

新职能

可见链接（荷兰）：该计划的目标是额外招募 150 名社区护士。2011 年春季中期审查期间，共有 95 个社区项目在 50 个城市中进行。当时，这些项目额外招募了约 355 名员工。其中 250 人为职业培训水平较高的社区护士（71%），75 名为中等职业水平的社区护士（20%），约 30 名为社区工作者等其他领域的员工。同时该计划也为项目经理创造了就业。鉴于中期审查期间，并非所有项目都完成征聘和甄选，"可见链接"计划的各社区护士和其他员工的最终数目一定会更多。

医护人员新职业（波兰）：没有可供使用的定量信息。

组织和指导照料工作的新方式

邻里照料（荷兰）：该计划始于 2006 年阿尔梅洛市的一个自我管理的社区团队。到 2012 年，该团队人员从 2011 年的 360 人达到 470 人。2012 年，社区团队的从业人员数达 5500 人，远高于 2011 年的 3700 人。每年平均招聘的员工约有 1200 人。

独立生活（西班牙）：这个区域性方案始于 2004 年，当时只涉及 4 个人。8 年后，有 39 人参加了该项计划。估计每个受益人平均产生 2 个或者 3 个个人助理职位，这表明创造的就业

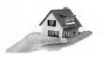

岗位数量是在 78—117 个之间。

SSI 集团（西班牙）：根据 2011 年度报告，SSI 集团共有 320 名员工。其中大多数（99%）是女性。截至 2012 年年底，集团总人数已增至 400—450 人。

科技创新

诺福克辅助技术（英国）：在过去几年间，AT 服务人员已从 6 名增至 13 名。原来的 6 名 AT 服务人员中，由于身体的缘故，有 1 人离开。由于辅助技术服务的引入，员工人数没有减少。

为成年残疾人提供的新型就业和交通服务

社会创业（保加利亚）：该方案的结果是建立了 29 个新的社会企业，其中 10 个已经得到了资助。2012 年该项目总人数为来自不同人群的 3612 人，其中 1606 人为残疾人。超过 140 人从事社会和医疗服务的交付（delivery）工作，这些工作主要是兼职和临时工作。

工作建立和服务支持（ESATs）（法国）：2001 年，ESATs 有 25500 名员工。2006 年，一共有 1345 个，ESATs 目前拥有 2.9 万名员工，为大约 11 万残疾人提供医疗，社会和就业支持。

PMR 交通服务（法国）：2007 年在 65 个主要城市进行的调查显示，PMR 交通服务雇用了 700 人，其中 80% 是司机。在巴黎，每年有超过 160 万次的旅行使用这些服务。

二 结论和影响

在对国别报告进行分析的基础上，可以得出有关这些举措的结果和影响的总体结论。

（1）在大多数情况下，这些举措的量化目标都已经达成或预计达成。所选择的方法也通常在实践中运作良好或者被证明至少是得当的。

（2）这些举措对劳动力市场产生积极的影响，有助于创造就业机会，招聘和留住雇员。同时，也解决了失业和员工短缺的问题。

（3）具有社会效益：这些举措有助于失业人员的社会融合，给予弱势公民权利和改善生活质量，并且还有助于社区内的凝聚力。

此外，正如国家报告中所示，大多数研究的举措都是预期或已经被证明是可持续的，并且可以转让给同一国家的其他组织或地区。有时候，这些举措已经被其他国家和组织采纳。

这些积极的成果部分应归于前文所述（PRESTLE 因素，如第 2 章所述），为社区照料提供了有利的环境，除此之外，当然也应归于举措本质特点和质量的原因（参见下一章关于成功与失败因素的讨论）。

第五章 经验教训：成功与失败的因素

本章专注于前两章讨论过的 30 个招聘和保留雇员措施的经验与教训。本章鉴别了与这些举措相关的成功和失败的因素，根据解决方案模型的四种对策，对这些因素进行分类和检验。除此之外，还会讨论这些措施的可持续性以及对其他地区、国家和行业可转让性的经验教训。

策略 1 的经验教训：以储备劳动力为目标
失业求职者就业计划

大多数欧洲国家都有健康和社会照料行业失业求职者的就业计划。这些计划为不同的利益相关者提供福利：失业人员可以获得有偿工作的必要资格证明；雇主可以聘请合格的雇员填补职位空缺；客户可以得到他们需要的照料服务。失业成本得以减少。

通常，这些项目包括提供职业培训或工作经验，或者两者兼有。在某些情况下，雇主也有劳务成本补贴。

招聘，选拔和资格预审

在失业的求职者接受培训之前，他们必须通过招募、选拔，有时候，通过多种方法进行资格预审。

（1）对于求职者，更适宜的招募不仅通过大规模的劳动力市场信息宣传活动，而且通过与求职者的个人协商来进行。

（2）优先考虑传统意义上碎片化的劳动力市场，例如，长期失业人员或具有种族背景的人员，这样有助于实现广泛的一体化目标。

（3）达到特定目标群体的劳动力储备，如移民人口，需要具体的有针对性的方法。在"移民照料"（奥地利）举措中，提供个人咨询（对移民的资格和动机进行评估，并对未来的工作领域进行实际的了解）被证明是一个重要的成功因素。

（4）社会工作和健康护理专业人员劳动基金会（奥地利）和单程票计划（英国）强调为失业求职者在就业计划中，提供一个好而谨慎的选拔程序的重要性，不仅要仔细挑选候选人，而且还要对未来的雇主进行筛选。

（5）失业求职者的财政激励可以消除参与就业计划的壁垒。例如，葡萄牙 EIP 计划的受益人可以获得增补款项，并保留其他补贴或福利。

职业培训

失业求职者的职业培训有以下这些成功和失败的因素。

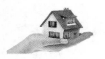

（1）好的职业培训机构就像好的申请求职者一样重要。在奥地利劳工基金会的举措中，对不同教育机构的成果进行比较监督。比较结果表明，较高的教育机构的质量对职业培训水平有很大帮助。

（2）使用正式规定的、公认的课程有助于雇主接纳员工。

（3）失业求职者的职业培训工作至关重要。例如，英国单程票计划由四个要素组成：独特的招聘流程；一个为期4周的就职入门训练；在健康与社会保健领域分别提供约为12周的5个单独的实习工作模块，预备5个不同工作背景的资料，为申请长期工作提供了坚实的基础；以及一个完成该计划的国家认可资格证书。求职者可以免费参加该计划，也被看作是一个成功的因素。在这种情况下，可能的失败因素包括需要参与者前往各种实习工作地点，找到足够的可以提供工作的组织机构，在这些合作组织内找到合适的了解该计划理念的人员，以及即将改变这些组织机构中的一些现有雇员的抵触情绪。

（4）许多案例显示，职业培训计划的参与者会事先确保有一份工作。有时，雇主也会了解未来的员工。这能激励候选人完成培训课程，同时，也意味着培训可以根据雇主的愿望和需求进行微调。

工作经验

获得工作经验也有助于提高失业求职者在劳动力市场中的机会。"工作轮岗"计划（丹麦）的成功因素就是事先为失业人员做工作面试、工作主管的指导，以及实习期结束后还能得到继续教育的保证。

调解和后续支持

当职业培训或工作实习在不能保证得到工作的情况下完成时，或者培训的候选人没有被事先承诺工作的雇主雇佣时，则需要进行调解。例如，奥地利劳工基金会计划有补充的安置服务。

在某些情况下，针对失业人员的就业项目会造成固定或兼职工作，这些处境似乎需要一些对新雇员的后续支持。然而，事实上，无法提供后续支持。

劳动力成本补贴

一般来说，雇主的经济激励措施，例如劳动力成本补贴，可能是一个有效的市场措施。通常，劳动力成本补贴的主要目标是为弱势求职者创造就业机会。葡萄牙的 2012 年激励计划并不要求雇主提供永久性雇佣合同，这可能会被看作此措施的主要成功因素。补贴额度对于雇主来说很划算，同时这也允许将此措施与其他措施相结合，有助于此举措的成功。

非正式就业正规化

案例研究还提供了以前非正式就业正规化的例子。例如，残疾人亲属可以申请加入保加利亚残疾人助理计划。独立生活计划（西班牙）使残疾人能够向个人助理提供合同，并且他们可以自己选择个人助理是否为亲戚。SSI 集团公司（西班牙）的明确目标之一就是使非正式照料者拥有资格证明，并以此提

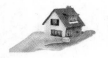
高其工作价值。

策略 2 的经验教训：鼓励和促进教育
活动和教育指导

在许多欧洲国家，广泛的运动旨在提高青年人关于照料行业及其课程和职业的认识。但是，具体问题需要具体分析。"男孩节"（奥地利）的成功因素包括在全国范围内针对当地的情况量身定制的举措，并且全年开展诸如市场营销、电影宣传和学校举办工作导向研讨会这样的活动，旨在维护男孩节最初的宗旨。这些研讨会被认定为男孩节最有效的影响因素。

德国展望未来计划表明，通过建立和维护本地或本区的社交网络，通过网络成员为培训课程提供的蓝图，可以完善社区照料行业专业化。

在这一举措中知识的成功转移依赖于同伴学习方式，让受训人员成为中学生的老师，再让学生在照料机构进行为期两周的实习。学习气氛轻松、无拘无束，便于大家讨论，同时，信息也会以一种幽默的方式呈现出来，从而轻松加强知识传送。

内容和教育设置

健康和社会照料的教育内容以及教学设置必须经过仔细研究。课程必须对相关学生有吸引力，但是，同时要适合未来雇主的需要。

就为工作学习而言，实践比理论更为重要。对于贫困学生，如移民和那些低学历的人，强化辅导和个人关注十分重要。

辅导具有种族背景的健康和社会照料学生（丹麦）的成功因素一是导师协调人网络，通过网络与学校联系和合作以获得学校的支持；二是学生和导师的正确匹配。双方的预期都要相似，而且年龄差距不能太大，如果他们年龄相近的话会更有帮助。其中一个失败的因素可能是导师缺乏足够的时间给学生提供咨询服务。

实习生职位

实习职位弥补了教育与劳动力市场的差距。有吸引力的实习岗位有助于激励学生的动力，并鼓励他们成功完成学业，进行更高层次的教育，或者选择社区照料行业入职。此外，他们有助于更好地配合教育机构提供的培训和雇主的要求。

以社区为基础，实习训练为主的荷兰邻里培训公司有一个很重要的成功因素，就是部署"劳工经纪人"，使学生与相符的客户匹配。

INOV-SOCIAL 措施（葡萄牙）的一个成功因素是社会照料行业的工作推销，通过提高学生对社会照料行业和机构的认识，给学生提供令他们感兴趣的学徒制。这一举措的失败因素则是相对较高的行政负担和成本。为了帮助年轻的毕业生进入劳动力市场，还会提供学徒培训，以及工资补贴，以减少雇主的劳动力成本。这可能会导致滥用这些措施来吸引实习生，而不考虑他们个人发展的需要。

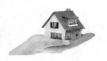

策略 3 的经验教训：改善现有雇员的环境

目前，以社区为基础照料员工的现状可能会通过行业专业化、员工资格和技能的提升而得到改善。这样做的方法包括在线学习的定期培训计划和专业认证。

行业专业化

以社区为基础的护理行业专业化，首要的是制订和提高在该行业工作和雇员的标准。比如，波兰使用社区组织模型，开发本国社会工作者的作用。

建立和维持伙伴关系，以发展行业劳动力为目标，可以促进区域和地方一级的行业专业化。SCWDOP（英国）框架下的合作伙伴关系就是一个很好的例子。然而，这里的一个失败因素是由于 SCWDP 作为私人供应商支持者，引发了对它作用的一些争议。但是，多年以来，私人资助的照料服务有所改变。现在大多数照料服务已经转包给独立的行业承包商，地方当局很少直接提供服务。

为专业的照料人员提供额外的管理技能，也有助于该行业的专业化。德国职业发展专业化举措将这实用的部分纳入课程，这成为一个关键的成功因素。这为在护理学校的人力资源顾问提供了进入照料服务管理的切入点，对提高社区照料专业化管理需求的认识产生了积极的效果。

员工培训

通过培训或再培训员工技能，提高了社区照料服务的质量。同时，有助于个人的职业发展和对工作的满意度。员工的管理新职责的信息越来越多，从而提高了员工的就业机会，也开辟了更多职业发展机会，使员工能够更上一层楼，收入更高。在有吸引力的环境下，再培训以社区为基础的雇员，不仅可以帮助他们的个人和职业发展，而且还有助于鼓励他们继续在该行业工作。

丹麦发展慢性病管理医护人员技能的重要成功因素在于客座教师是从实际工作环境中部署的，课程以实践为导向。其他成功因素还有小班授课（允许参与者与其他部门进行对话沟通），定期评估和持续满足学员对课程的需求和愿望。一个失败的因素与该计划选择跨部门操作方式有关，难以区分课程以满足不同行业参与者的具体需求。

保加利亚的社会助理和家庭助理服务补助金计划则旨在通过介绍培训、支持培训和监督来提高社会助理和家庭助理的技能和积极性。这种计划方式最后成为一个成功因素。

波兰提高照料人员资格的措施也表明拥有吸引力且充分的的培训设置的重要性。成功因素包括有现代设备场所的课程，以及有专业且热情的护理人员帮助激励参与者。参加培训的阻碍可能是培训成本和抵达培训设施场所的差旅费。

一般来说，员工更愿意在工作时间内进行训练。对于雇主来说，这可能是一个阻碍，因为在工作时间接受培训的员工效率不高。工作轮岗制度（丹麦）解决了这个问题，让失业人员暂时接手了正在接受培训的员工的工作。

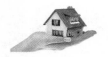

专业经验认证

专业经验认证可以被定义为通过工作经验或非正式的培训方式获得知识、技能和能力的一种机制，并且有专业证书可以认证。例如，西班牙的专业证书计划和基于法国工作经验的专业认证体系。这两个计划都促进了社区照料行业的专业化，提高了员工的资质，同时，也促进了劳动力市场在行业中的流通，从而明确了其员工所掌握的技能。在法国系统中，与传统职业培训相比，工作经验认证成本相对较低，因为雇员在工作培训时是有生产力的，这被认定是一个重要的成功因素。而一个失败因素则是笔试的评估程序。更实际的测试方法无疑可以让更多具有较弱写作能力的候选人受益，系统的专业支持也将提高认证程序的成功率。

在线学习

在线学习（使用网络连接的计算机的互动式培训）具有成本优势。在社区照料行业支持开发在线学习的其他主要理由包括：雇员职业和继续教育的更多选择；灵活性；轻松适应个人学习步骤；减少路上时间和费用；对年轻人的吸引力。

第二章（CARICT）描述的研究项目对这些论点给予了支持。

照料行业的在线学习计划（德国）显示，在雇主的设施中，有足够数量的智能终端有助于在线学习的成功。这也表明，离传统教育设施越远，在线学习就越容易被接受。一个失败因素则是，年长的决策者和老师可能会对在线学习持怀疑态度，他们与年轻人相比，对电子媒体的熟悉程度较低。

策略 4 的经验教训：提高经营管理水平和劳动生产率

除了降低劳动力成本外，通过新的工作方式提高运营管理和劳动生产率，有助于吸引以社区为基础的照料行业现有和潜在的员工，从而改善招聘和保留雇员的条件。

功能创新

创建新类型的功能可以提高以社区为基础的照料工作的效率。一种可行方式是"job carving"，这是一种工作分工，各尽所能的方式，以确保用最适合的人员来执行每项任务。这样可以创造新的工作机制。这是一种灵活的管理劳动力的方式，允许员工各尽所能，这使能力不强的工作人员（如残疾人）也能够为工作做出宝贵的贡献。在波兰，通过在官方名单中登记注册医护新职业，促进了这一举措的成功。

另一种提高社区照料工作的效率和吸引力的方法是令该领域的专业人员更富有责任感和自主权。荷兰"可见链接"计划推出的新型社区护士增加了更多的协调性职能，也加强了这些卫生专业人员的主观能动性，这对现有员工来说是非常有吸引力的。

组织创新

通过改变照料管理活动的组织或管理，例如，应用自我指导区域团队和合作社等观念，以加强社区照料的运作。

像荷兰的邻里照料计划那样的自我指导团队运作良好的前

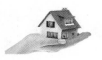

提条件包括：（1）团队在一定条件下自己做出决定并且赞同管理的能力；（2）团队协调平衡，内部关系良好并且可以互相协商任务分工；（3）以解决问题为导向的定期讨论工作会议，决策在讨论中达成一致；（4）对组织任务和成果的共同责任，同时，明确谁、何时可以防止队员工作负担过重，尤其是在计划阶段。

SSI集团（西班牙）的合作模式的特点是自我管理、集体参与并且共享所有权，交流合作以及权力下放的人力资源结构。其他基本价值观念则体现为个人成长、发展专业精神以及培养社会主动性。这个合作模式是SSI成功的主要因素。

直接支付计划使客户有效地成为其照料人员的雇主，同时也改变了传统的照料服务组织。西班牙独立生活计划的研究案例说明了这一方法的成败因素。关于该计划管理和运作的成功因素包括：（1）通过"行动议定书"对受益人的具体需求进行微调，并且对这些需求进行充分的评估，使他们花在照料上的钱更加合理；（2）确保客户与个人助理之间直接达成协议，没有地方当局干涉；（3）制订应急措施来应对特殊情况，例如，没有任何个人助理有空工作的情况。

如果没有雇用亲属或朋友，并且有几名兼职助理而不是一名全职助理，那么成功招聘和调度个人助理的可能性似乎会更大。助理需要知道的是，残疾人有能力做出自己的决定，反过来，"雇主"需要从一开始就明确规定助理要做的任务。在理想情况下，可以制订出"独立生活计划"，可以充分描述所有的照料和帮助需求，以便确定个人助理的工作内容。最后，如果方案的受益人可以组织起来相互支持并且分享经验教训将会是很有益的。

技术创新

通过在家里提供创新的技术支持系统，可以改善社区照料的运作，帮助残疾人和老年人在自己家中居住。技术解决方案往往更具成本效益，可以有效地为社会和健康提供支持。科技也减少了相对稀缺的健康和社会照料工作人员的需要。

这已经得到 CARICT 项目的证实。非正式护理人员的技术服务的调度和使用仍然有限，主要是由于使用者的对数字技能的掌握是有限的，在现实生活中缺少此类服务的实例以及这些服务的影响和可持续性的证据。该项目旨在基于收集在家中 ICT-照料服务影响的结果证据，并提出制订、扩大和复制欧盟的政策建议。该方法基于在欧洲发展的非正式护理人员的 52 个 ICT 的服务项目筹划和 12 项举措的交叉分析，以便收集有关其影响、驱动因素、商业模式、成功因素和挑战的数据。主要结果表明，在欧洲各地的护理人员中，有许多 ICT 成功但成本不高的例子。交叉分析表明，这些服务对老年人和非正式护理人员的生活质量、照料质量、健康与社会保健系统的财务可持续性产生了积极的影响。

诺福克辅助技术计划（英国）的重要成功因素包括对组织内举措的支持，定期增强服务意识和培训，以人为本的理念，由 AT 人员提供针对个人需求量身定做的设备。该计划也遇到

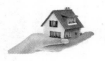

一些障碍，其障碍有四点：①社会服务专业人士在组织内的态度，他们中的一些人把辅助技术视为附加服务而不是核心服务；②组织内存在一种假设：老年人不理解新技术；③临床医生认为这些服务对他们的工作构成威胁；④对有技能的雇员任命和管理系统缺乏正式资格认可。

残疾成年人就业服务

残疾人就业服务不仅旨在引导他们找到有报酬的工作，而且是正规劳动市场中的工作，并且还要在他们工作时继续给予支持。在本报告研究的一些案例中，残疾人与长期失业人员、老年失业人员和移民人口等其他群体形成了一个特定的就业计划目标群体。

社会企业会通过积极参与劳动力市场的方式来提供就业机会，提升包括残疾人在内的弱势群体的生活质量和社会融入。保加利亚社会创业补助金计划的研究案例表明，企图通过社会企业刺激就业时可能会出现一些失败因素，比如，经济危机，会导致对社会企业服务需求的减少，以及公众社会意识的缺乏和访问目标群体的困难。

现在针对把残疾人安置到正规劳动力市场上的"残疾友好型"公司里的政策越来越多，如有必要的话，会有工作指导支持。虽然许多欧洲国家继续支持受庇护的工作环境，但是这只适用于无法在正常劳动力市场上工作的成年人。

法国 ESATs 面临的一个问题就是他们会相互竞争。政府提高效率的要求可能会产生负面影响，继而推动 ESATs 只接受生产能力较高的残疾人士，从而减少在工作中效率较低的雇员人数。某些 ESATs 设施很难适应更好的绩效和更专业化的管理需求。在未来，一旦国家补贴不足以达到收支平衡，有些人将遭遇生存困境。

残疾成年人运输服务

特殊运输服务使得不方便移动的成年残疾人能够积极参与社会活动，例如，可以将他们运送到教育或工作场所。许多公共交通系统正在努力为残疾人提供更好的无障碍环境，但仍然还存在一些问题，问题突出地表现在残疾人从家庭到公共交通系统的行程中。该服务向行动不方便的人提供额外的特殊运输服务，帮助他们定期或偶尔地从家到达目的地，通过专门的车辆和司机护理人员，满足残疾人的交通需求，帮助他们融入社会。

法国格勒诺布尔的 PMR 运输服务以社会照料、培训能为残疾成人提供运输服务的驾驶员为工作。这项服务是成功的，其乘客人数和司机护理人员的就业人数正在稳步增加。其成功的因素包括，公共成本削减和医务运输授权的减少，有限活动能力下能够独立生活的人口数量增加。

吸取经验：可持续性和可转让性

在护理机构中，成功招聘和保留雇员措施的可持续性是重要的，将成功举措的经验用于其他领域情况也一样。从研究的30 个不同的案例中，可以得出若干关于招聘和保留雇员措施的

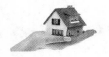

可持续性和可转让性的综合观察结果。

可持续发展

（1）政治和公众支持

制定政策和将资源用于照料行业的政治意愿是可持续性的关键因素。虽然这似乎是不言而喻的，但政治行为在很大程度上植根于选民对提议政策的重要性如何看待。当舆论在一个特定政策方向中看到价值时，将资源用于该政策就是合法的。

就照料工作而言，一些案例研究的是有关政府对继续支持新政策的意愿和动机的重要性。因此，如果政治利益是想增加并促进照料行业的可持续性，那么确保公众意识到照料行业日益增长的需求，以及照料行业在社会中扮演着越来越重要的角色是非常重要的。

一些措施试图做到这一点。奥地利男孩节旨在宣传医疗保健这份有价值和有益的职业，同时，也为人们提供照料行业日益增长的雇员需求信息。德国照料未来计划有非常类似的目标。

在其他国家，则需要改变对残疾人照料和老年人照料的态度。例如，在保加利亚，如果在家照顾弱势的亲戚则会被认为是对家庭成员的义务，这限制了他们的工作自由，降低了社区照料的政策数量以及从制度化到社区照料的转移率。然而，随着各种关心弱势群体心态的出现，这种现象开始趋于缓和。在西班牙也有类似情况：对照顾残疾人或老年亲属的态度正在逐渐改变。社区照料被认为是整个社会必须为之努力的问题。西班牙独立生活计划表明了政治意愿在维持这一措施中的重要性。在波兰，对社会保健的新态度重振了照料行业。

（2）资金

可持续性措施的第二个关键因素是要有充足的资金。本报告中的大多数案例研究表明，资金来自各个公共机构，如市政府、国家机关和 ESF。在一些情况下，这些措施与受益方的贡献相结合，无论是公司、小型社会保健医疗机构还是客户。无论如何，大部分举措都需要公共部门的财政补贴。鉴于目前欧洲的经济环境，带来了能否持续发展的问题。这意味着继续资助这些项目的政治意愿是至关重要的。

一些国家正在遭遇这个特别的问题。在德国、丹麦和保加利亚，资金的不确定性是可持续发展的阻碍。在德国，eLiP 的倡议举措是自筹资金（自我维持），因为信息网络的成员都会支付一定费用。然而，大多数措施需要投入更多的财务支持，而且那种自筹资金的措施可能更加难以制订。

（3）合作与协作

可持续性受到存在或缺席两个息息相关的因素的影响：个人和有关组织之间有效的合作和协调。

在规划和实施措施中，所有相关参与者的观点都是重要的，因此组织的专业知识和见解会被纳入举措。这将最大限度地增强措施的影响和所涉及的人的满意度。最终既利于服务提供者又利于受益者的有效措施才更有可能持续下去。这一点在各国都是明显的，丹麦、法国和西班牙的案例研究尤其表明了

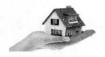

这种合作的重要性。

一种促进协同合作的具体手段则是建立信息和通信网络。一些案例研究证明了创建客户信息数据库的价值和实用性，以此来促进有关组织之间有效的协作。

荷兰邻里照料计划使用信息技术基础设施来报告和计划照料人员的到访和任务。德国 eLiP 项目围绕共享 IT 网络的概念，促进照料人员之间互相学习。西班牙的专业证书依靠汇集了有关各机构和政府机关的客户信息的数据库，尽可能高效地颁发资格证书。保加利亚则使用一种促进与客户更好沟通的残疾人助理项目系统，大大减少了提供给残疾人的照料潜在的低效率和失败因素。

可转让性

当涉及源于该地区措施的可转让性时，必须考虑到国家现有的社会支持和医疗体系。例如，在法国，残疾人受益于一些改善社会照料方面的重要津贴；但是单靠这些措施不可能在其他国家给予残疾人足够的支持。波兰的观察数据也同样表明，任何措施的成功取决于是否在法律和政治的框架里开展运作。

然而，在原籍国转让措施似乎问题不大。一些案例研究表明，可以将措施转让到一个国家的不同地区和城市，或者不同的照料或劳动环境。同一个国家的不同地区对社会保健和医疗卫生的需求可能不同，因此，劳动力供求水平将会有所不同。但是，适应这些因素还是可行的。

大多数案例研究表明，所描述的措施可以转移到不同的情况中。保加利亚的社会创业补助金计划可以转移到具有不同级别的残疾或照料需求的目标群体中；丹麦的工作轮岗计划和留学生指导都可以应用于劳动力市场的不同群体中；波兰的提高护理人员资格的措施也可适用于其他职业；奥地利男孩节已经被其他职业所运用；荷兰邻里培训公司计划也可为在其他行业中的年轻人提供经验。

一些举措可能会跨越国界进行转移，因为它们的法律和政治框架更为简单。例如，葡萄牙大多数案例研究使用最简单的补贴，所以，在其他国家政治允许的情况下，INOV-SOC 和 2012 年刺激计划可以相对轻松地实施。奥地利的"男孩节"已经在德国实施。荷兰邻里照料的理念也已经在其他国家实施，因为它不依赖于其他社会照料和医疗保健的组合。

第六章　结论与政策指向

　　本研究的中心内容是针对以社区为基础照料的残疾或患有疾病的成年人的创造就业、招聘和保留问题。一个运作良好、可持续发展和高质量的社区健康和社会照料供给对欧洲社会和经济至关重要。同时，这个行业提供了很多就业机会。为了克服该行业创造就业的阻碍，如预算限制和苛刻的工作条件等。同时，为了支持在该行业中建立强大且不断增长的劳动力队伍，许多国家已经采取不同的招聘和保留雇员措施。本研究探讨了10个不同国家有益实践的30个案例，以便其他国家学习。

一　结论

　　在研究的10个国家中，与非机构照料服务相比，照料残疾成年人的机构比例千差万别。然而，非机构照料服务越来越多。

趋向家庭照料发展的趋势则是由成本降低、帮助残疾人独立的政策、客户的偏好以及辅助生活技术的潜在动力所带来的。

一般来说，为残疾成年人提供服务的照料和支援行业的劳动力市场雇员短缺，尤其缺少较高资格水平的人员。从照料人员本身来看，在资质上面存在差异，因为他们的就业待遇和工作条件一般不好。这个行业存在形象问题，部分原因是就业待遇差和工作环境不好这样的客观性问题，还有一部分原因在于主观感受，认为照料行业的职业地位不高。

目前，由于经济危机，劳动力短缺的问题暂时得到缓解。从长远来看，随着人口数量的增长和欧洲经济的复苏，劳动力供给会下降，然而长期照料的需求会持续上升，预计会出现供不应求的现象。科技创新的发展可能导致家庭照料中劳动生产率的提高，但此行业仍将是劳动密集型。

为了防止上述劳动力市场差异，所研究的案例基本都确定了四项总体战略：①以劳动力储备为目标；②促进和提升潜在雇员的教育；③改善现有员工的环境；④提高组织的经营管理水平和劳动生产率。

所研究的 10 个国家在这些类别中都有举措，虽然侧重点有所不同。本报告共记录和评估了 30 项创新性方法，所有实施的方法都被证明对招聘和留住家庭照料人员是有用的。在这四个劳动力市场战略中的每一个领域，可以选择不同类型的项目。它们包括：①劳动储备—职业定位，资格和资格预审，工作经验，调解或后续支持，劳务成本补贴；②教育—劳动力市

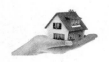

场传播活动和教育或职业导向，健康和社会照料方面的学徒制，导师制；③现有员工——行业专业化，培训和再培训计划，培养和教育人才的新方法，如在线学习和凭经验专业资格认证等；④运营管理和劳动生产率——新功能，组织和指导照料活动新方式，技术创新，新的就业和运输服务。

一般来说，这30个案例研究的结果和结论都是很有前途的。这些措施在劳动力市场具有积极的影响，例如，促进创造就业机会，招聘或者留住雇员。同时，还带来一些社会效益，因为许多措施有助于失业人员的社会包容，或者赋予弱势公民权利，提升他们的生活质量以及邻里间的社会凝聚力。最终，研究的多数举措都已被证明是可持续的，也可以转让给同一国家的其他组织或地区。有时候，转移到其他国家也是可行的，而且已有一些成功案例。

二 政策指向

对这30项个案研究的分析，确定了招聘和留住家庭照料人员的一些成功和失败因素。基于分析，本研究提出了一系列与四个劳动力市场策略相关的方针政策，以及关于可持续性和可转移性的成功举措以及一些更为普遍的政策方针。

（一）以劳动力储备为目标

家庭照料服务可为长期失业人员、流动人口和残疾成年人提供就业机会。以流动人口和残疾成年人为目标的人群得到特别的关注。在一些欧洲国家，相当多数量的移民已经在非正式照料行业拥有相关的工作经验。家庭照料行业中将残疾成年人作为有实际经验的专家会提升附加值，因为他们与服务用户感同身受。

（1）达到不同群体的劳动力储备需要一种具体、量身定做的，明确目标群体的方法。

（2）失业求职者必须免费参与就业计划，并且可以保留其他补贴或福利，财政奖励可激励求职者参与该就业计划。

（3）适当的选拔程序有助于失业求职者就业计划的成功。在家庭照料行业工作的承诺和意愿可以视为正式资格认定的重要标准。语言障碍必须通过资格预审培训来消除。

（4）潜在的员工必须仔细选择，未来的雇主也必须如此；劳动力市场供需双方应当匹配。

（5）通过质量措施（使用官方规定，认可的课程和教育机构之间质量对比）和适当的培训组织（参与者在地域上与实习基地和工作安置都比较临近），确保和增强失业求职人员培训的效果。

（6）强烈推荐事先保证一份工作的举措。这将鼓励参与者完成培训课程，这也意味着培训可以根据雇主的愿望和需求进行调整。

（7）为了促进更广泛就业能力，职业培训参与者应较好地完成在该行业各部门的工作实习。

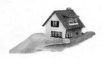

（8）已经合格的失业求职者获得的工作经验会增加他们在劳动力市场的就业机会。

（9）如有需要，失业求职者在成功完成工作计划后必须通过调节服务和后续支持来寻找工作和保留工作。劳动力成本补贴可以诱使雇主雇用他们。

（二）鼓励和促进教育

（1）如果针对特定群体的话，鼓励年轻人考虑在照料行业工作的活动会更为成功。在这方面，使用角色模型增加附加值。说服男孩选择照料工作是一项有成效的职业，任重而道远。这种活动应该是结构化的和持续性的，全年应有"活动日"或"活动周"。在这方面，专业导向课程，特别是由地区或区域网络组织的，遵循同伴互相学习方法，包括在照料机构实习的，是一项很有效的手段。

（2）健康和社会护理教育（包括实习生职位）的内容和组织必须对有关学生有吸引力，同时适应未来雇主的愿望和需要。这意味着要强调实践经验、在职培训、集中辅导和个人关注。这特别有益于由教师或护理人员指导教育水平较低的贫困学生和移民。

（3）实习生职位弥合了照料教育与劳动力市场之间的差距。对于不很符合资格的学生来说，以社区为基础的实践训练是一个很好的办法，在这种训练中学生会被指定一位由当地居民担任的"劳动经纪人"。

（4）除了实习作为他们学习的一部分之外，高水平毕业生的专业学徒制将巩固他们的专业技能，并且可以促进他们融入社会护理劳动力市场。为了不让雇主滥用专业学徒制，补贴不应太高。

（三）改善员工现状

（1）为了缩小照料服务工作的供求差距，改善工作条件和就业条件，必须得到社会合伙人和其他有关组织的长期关注。

（2）社区照料行业专业化需要制订和提高该部门工作和员工的标准。为了在地方一级适当实施这些标准，建立和维护公共和私人双方的伙伴关系，负责开发、规划、监测和评估整体家庭照料劳动力的培训是有帮助的。现有的护理人员可以接受培训来承担额外的管理任务。

（3）培训或再培训雇员最理想的是与相关参与者地理位置接近，并在工作时间内，报销交通费用和其他费用。在配备现代化设施场地进行实习时，与实践经验丰富的客座老师交流，也会增效和更具吸引力。小班授课是很重要的，课程的定期评估以及课程适应参与者的愿望和需求同样也都是重要的。与来自不同社区的照料和职业工作者的跨部门培训，也有助于思想和经验的交流学习，并且导致以社区为基础照料的更综合的方法。同时，也提高参与者的就业能力。

（4）工作轮岗制可以弥补经历漫长培训或再培训的员工的缺位，他们会暂时由具有合适的专业资格并获得工作经验的失

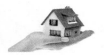

业人员代替。

（5）传统的员工培训方式应该与获取资格证书的现代方式相补充，凭借经验和在线学习确认特别的专业验证。鼓励具有较低资格水平的人员进行资格验证时，需要基于更多的实际评估，而不是基于书面测试。为学生提供专业支持会提高成功率。根据该行业量身定做的在线学习系统可以增强他们的接受和使用。

（四）提高经营管理和劳动生产率

（1）功能差异化或分工合作可以适用于家庭照料工作，因为这有助于提高效率，降低在高资质水平上员工的工作压力，并使弱势群体如残疾成年人参与劳动力市场。同时，带给员工更多的责任感，使该行业的工作更有吸引力。这可以通过增强协调或任务管理的行政职能来实现；或者通过创建自我指导的团队；也可以通过鼓励自我管理来实现。

（2）直接支付系统的发展空间很大，客户会成为个人助理的雇主。适当的直接支付制度的先决条件包括根据受益人的具体需要进行调整，简化其行政管理，并确保在个人助理不可用的意外情况下采取紧急措施。

（3）通过使用专业人员来评估潜在用户的愿望和需求，协助生活技术的接受和使用，如家庭自动化和远程监护已经得到了完善。这些专业人员可以安装设备，同时也为用户和其他有关人员提供培训。

（4）残疾成年人就业服务，比如，遮蔽工作间和公众工作场合，可以提高弱势群体的生活质量以及帮助他们融入社会。可能的话，庇护工作的员工应该在正规劳动力市场中工作，无论是残疾人友好型公司还是"正常"公司。在工作中，由就业指导员支持他们可以提升他们在正常劳动力市场的工作能力。

（5）在社会照料行业受过培训的驾驶员，会对残疾成年人人士提供更好的交通服务。

三　可持续性和可转移性的政策指向

就补贴项目，可持续性举措值得特别注意。项目结束后，必须找到替代资金，确保项目管理的协调活动，确定发挥主导作用的一方。

成功转移举措到其他环境（其他地区、国家或行业）需要深入考虑主流化战略。[①] 这样的策略需要关注消息的接受者（接近哪位决策者以及如何接近）；定时传播消息（何时接近决策者）；消息的内容（要宣传哪些具体消息）；消息的形式（使用什么工具向决策者传递消息）。[②]

----

① 主流化可以定义为在相同或其他情况下将成功的创新嵌入常规活动或政策。

② 2007 年，Panteia 定制了一份主流化项目成果手册，见 Ministry of van Sociale Zaken en Wergelegenheid，2007。

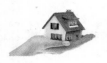

四　基本政策方针

第一，在家庭照料中防止劳动力市场短缺的各种策略都有自己的优点。鉴于它们的互补性，把这些策略措施以综合方法相连是可行的。

第二，在欧洲，家庭照料的需求预计在未来几年会有明显增加。这就需要加大劳动力市场的政策力度。在照料和支持服务行业中，招聘和保留雇员需要解决的问题包括不太有利的就业条件，如工资低，工作条件差，工作时间长，公众形象不好。除国家政策外，社会合伙人达成的集体协议可以在解决这些问题上发挥重要作用。

第三，在一些国家，必须改变对照顾残疾人和老年人的文化态度。特别是改变家庭成员只能在家照料的想法，这可能会限制家庭成员从事有偿就业的能力。增加社区服务不但有助于改善残疾人的独立性，而且也有助于提高其家庭生活质量。

第四，客户和机构作为需求方需要得到更多的关注。鉴于政府通常决定该行业的预算，这需要对客户的愿望和需求以及相关的政治发展情况进行摸底。

第五，"思考小的方面"，并在本地区区域运营的项目中创造灵活性，这可以帮助将新系统嵌入整个家庭照料系统中。这可以是自上而下的，将大规模的全国性计划适当地转化为区域和地方项目，或由自下而上，将区域性的和地方的实验项目在全国范围按比例扩大。

第六，劳动力市场举措的成功，特别是在照料行业，取决于与国家、地区或有关地方部门的合作、协调和承诺。

第七，"合适的人在正确的地方"是一个重要的成功因素，因为个人特性、项目经理的能力、所涉及合作者以及他们之间的私下交往的性质，可成事亦可败事。

第八，充分规划举措是必要的。必须监测和评估进展情况和结果。然而，同时也要尽可能避免官僚主义和行政负担。

第九，照料行业的需求正在增加，政治和公众的支持也是至关重要的。特别是在目前的经济环境下，健康与社会照料行业的价值和需求的重要性必须要向社会传播。信息和意识提升的活动是非常有用的，但这些活动需要长期的保证，因为它们需要时间才会产生效果。

第十，这个行业的成功劳动力市场举措有一个非常重要的先决条件，就是要拥有足够的结构性资金。

最后但同样重要的是，数据收集和使用统计数据，可以充分地改善、发展、监督、评估和调整国家和欧洲当局相关的劳动力市场政策。

参考文献[*]

1. Andor, L. (2011), We Care, How can the EU Care?, Conference Presentation, Social Platform's Annual Conference on Care, 9 December, Brussels.

2. Carretero, S., Stewart, J., Centeno, C., Barbabella, F., Schmidt, A., Lamontagne-Godwin, F. and Lamura, G. (2013), Can Technology-Based Services Support Long-term Care Challenges in Home Care? Analysis of Evidence from Social Innovation Good Practices across the EU, CARICT project summary report, Joint Research Centre of the European Commission, Publications Office of the European Union, Luxembourg.

3. Cedefop (European Centre for the Development of Vocational

---

* All Eurofound publications are available at www. eurofound. europa. eu.

Training）（2012），The Role of Qualifications in Governing Occupations and Professions, Cedefop, Thessaloniki.

4. EHMA（European Health Management Association）（2012），
EHMA's Workforce Taskforce Discussion Paper: Building a
Shared Agenda for Tackling Workforce Challenges, EHMA, Brus-
sels.

5. Eurofound（2006），Employment in Social Care in Europe, Publications Office of the European Union, Luxembourg.

6. European Commission（2006），The Impact of Ageing on Public
Expenditure: Projections for the EU25 Member States on Pen-
sions, Health Care, Long-term Care, Education and Unemployment
Transfers（2004 – 2050），Special Report No. 1/2006, Economic
Policy Committee and the Directorate-General of Economic and
Financial Affairs, Brussels.

7. European Commission（2007），Health and Long-term Care in the
European Union, Special Eurobarometer 283, European Commission, Brussels.

8. European Commission（2010），Second Biennial Report on Social
Services of General Interest, SEC（2010）1284 final, Brussels.

9. European Commission（2010），Europe 2020: A Strategy for
Smart, Sustainable and Inclusive Growth, COM（2010）2020 final, Brussels.

10. European Commission（2011），The Social Dimension of the Eu-

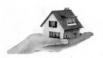 更多更好的家庭照料服务就业

rope 2020 Strategy: A Report of the Social Protection Committee, Publications Office of the European Union, Luxembourg.

11. European Commission (2012), Commission Staff Working Document on an Action Plan for the EU Health Workforce, SWD (2012) 93 final, Strasbourg.

12. European Commission (2012), Commission Staff Working Document on Exploiting the Employment Potential of the Personal and Household Services, SWD(2012) 95 final, Strasbourg.

13. European Commission (2012), Taking Forward the Strategic Implementation Plan of the European Innovation Partnership on Active and Healthy Ageing, COM(2012) 83 final, Brussels.

14. European Commission (2012), Towards a Job-rich Recovery, COM(2012) 173 final, Brussels.

15. European Commission (2012), The 2012 Ageing Report: Economic and Budgetary Projections for the 27 EU Member States (2010 – 2060), European Commission, Brussels.

16. European Commission (2013), Long-term Care in Ageing Societies—Challenges and Policy Options, SWD (2013) 41 final, Brussels.

17. European Commission (2013), Social Investment: Commission Urges Member States to Focus on Growth and Social Cohesion, press release, 20 February.

18. Ewijk, van H., Hens, H., and Lammersen, G. (2002), Map-

ping of Care Services and the Care Workforce: Consolidated Report, Working Paper No. 3, Thomas Coram Research Unit, Institute of Education, University of London.

19. Genet, N., Boerma, W., Kroneman, M., Hutchinson, A., and Saltman, R. B. (eds.) (2012), Home Care across Europe: Current Structure and Future Challenges, Observatory Studies No. 27, World Health Organization, Copenhagen.

20. Huber, M. (2007), Monitoring Long-term Care in Europe: Background Paper on Care Indicators, European Centre for Social Welfare Policy and Research, Vienna.

21. Korczyk, S. (2004), Long-term Workers in Five Countries: Issues and Options, AARP Public Policy Institute, Washington DC.

22. Lethbridge, J. (2012), Care Home versus Home Care? Which Direction for Care Services in Europe? Eligibility for European Works Councils, EPSU, Brussels.

23. Matrix Insight (2012), EU Level Collaboration on Forecasting Health Workforce Needs, Workforce Planning and Health Workforce Trends—A Feasibility Study, European Commission Executive Agency for Health and Consumers, Luxembourg.

24. Ministerie van Sociale Zaken en Werkgelegenheid [Netherlands Ministry for Social Affairs] (2007), Verknopen van innovaties. Handleiding voor mainstreaming van projectresultaten

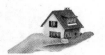

[Crosslinking innovations: Manual for mainstreaming of project results], Institute of Policy Research.

25. OECD (2011), Health at a Glance 2011-OECD Indicators, OECD Publishing, Paris.

26. OECD (2011), Help Wanted? Providing and Paying for Long-term Care, OECD Publishing, Paris.

27. Panteia, SEOR and Etil (2013), Effectmeting van arbeidsmarktmaatregelen in de zorgsector. Een haalbaarheidsstudie [Effects of labour market measures in the healthcare sector: A feasibility study], Panteia, Zoetermeer, the Netherlands.

28. Rodrigues, R., Huber, M. and Lamura, G. (eds.) (2012), Facts and Figures on Healthy Ageing and Long-term Care, European Centre for Social Welfare Policy and Research, Vienna.

附录 1　分析框架

在这项研究中，使用了三个模型来提供一个分析框架：

一是劳动力市场模型，绘制了劳动力供需现状和预期情况，并表明了供需矛盾。

二是 PESTLE 分析，描述了影响劳动力市场的外部因素（见图 A1）。

三是解决方案模型，针对解决劳动力市场问题的措施进行分类。

这些模型为研究具体问题，收集和分析数据以及报告调查结果打下了基础。

劳动力市场模型

劳动力市场政策的关键目标是发现供求平衡。如果不能满足需求，那么这个行业的潜能就得不到开发。如果劳动力

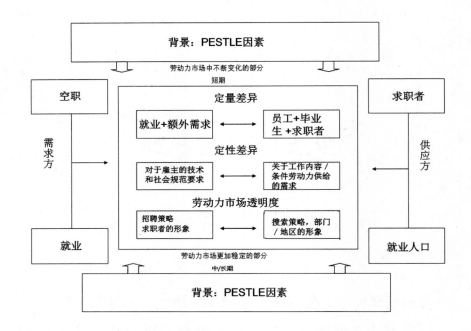

图 A1　在 PESTLE 因素背景下的劳动力市场模型

资料来源：Panteia

过剩，人们最后会以不适合的工作或者失业告终。理想的情况是要有一个动态平衡，从而可以适应该行业的潜在变化和发展，创造灵活且可持续的制度。许多部门和国家在劳动力市场上面临着供需矛盾。本报告涉及社区照料的具体情况，不匹配情况普遍并有可能更明显，其原因是人口总数一直在变化。这种劳动力市场差异具有定量或定性，也可以归结为缺乏透明度的劳动力市场组织形式。权衡供需可以指出存在的差异。

PESTLE 分析

外部因素影响劳动力市场的发展。这些因素可能给劳动力市场管理带来挑战或创造解决方案。可以通过查看 PESTLE 分析的六个具体方面来确定发展。

这六个具体方面分别是政治、经济、社会、技术、法律和环境。PESTLE 分析最初是一种商业模式，用于描述宏观层面的相关因素框架，主要用于分析组织的商业环境。它是衡量外部因素优势与劣势的方式，可以帮助组织制订战略。同样，PESTLE 分析也可以用于劳动力市场行业的情境分析。

这六个方面可能会对劳动力市场行业产生很大的影响，尽管这六个方面重要程度各不相同。在研究问题的背景下，政治和经济两方面必须重点考虑，因为它们会直接影响到社区照料行业创造有吸引力和有用的工作的可能性。在这里，财政方面也是特别重要的，因为照料行业不是一个普通的商业部门，而是一个通常用公共资金资助的行业。

由于本报告审查了不同国家的情况，与 PESTLE 相关的劳动力市场差异模型有助于快速确定每个国家的问题。该模型在某种意义上用通用语言描述为不同行为者所面临的挑战。由于以前的研究已经表明，该行业劳动力普遍短缺，有时候又缺乏就业机会，预计各个国家在这方面会有明显差异。该模型可以快速记录是否为定性或是定量，因为流出该行业的人流量远超流入该行业的人流量，这或许是由其中一

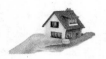

个 PESTLE 方面的发展而引起的。同时，该模型还提供了一种结构化的比较方法。

解决方案模型

PESTLE 模型缩小了挑战和解决方案之间的差距，并通向该研究的核心目标，即，确定可用于招聘和留住分派到以社区为基础的照料服务雇员的工具。

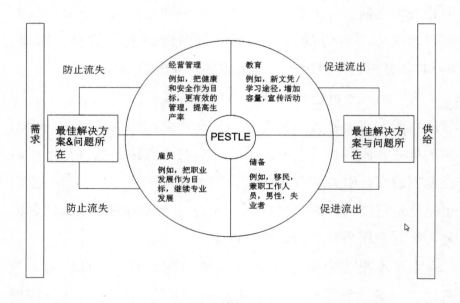

图 A2　解决方案模型

资料来源：Panteia

通过区分刺激劳动力供给的手段和缓解劳动力需求的手段，可以对潜在的解决方案进行分类，形成以下四项策略。

（1）以劳动力储备为目标，吸引新雇员进入该行业。

（2）促进和提升潜在雇员的教育。

（3）改善现有员工的现状，发挥他们最大的潜能，同时，预防员工离开该行业。

（4）提高该行业组织的运作管理和劳动生产率。

之前研究确定的大多数工具可以归类到象限中的其中一个，同时，也可作为专门减轻来自 PESTLE 因素之一的负面影响的工具。

附录 2　各国专家

本研究框架范围内的国家和个案研究是由欧洲社会经济研究网（ENSR）的各国专家在 Panteia 的监督下进行的，基于他们的参与，Panteia 草拟了这个综述报告。

ENSR 是一个专门从事应用社会和经济政策研究的机构网络，成立于 1991 年，由 EIM 商业与政策研究（现为 Panteia 的一部分）组成。ENSR 网络在欧盟 27 国的所有国家，以及挪威，冰岛，瑞士（也包括列支敦士登）和候选国土耳其都有代表。ENSR 涵盖共计 32 个国家。

以下 ENSR 专家参与了这项研究。

表 A1

国家	研究所	姓名
奥地利	奥地利中小企业研究所	英格里德·佩克
保加利亚	创业发展基金会	埃琳娜·克拉斯滕诺娃
丹麦	牛津集团	海勒·厄罗·尼尔森
法国	生存条件学习观察研究中心	艾萨·阿尔代
德国	中小企业研究所	弗兰克·马斯马丽娜·霍夫曼
荷兰	Panteia 咨询机构	道维·格里普斯特拉，彼得·德克拉沃，贾克林·斯内德斯，安伯·范德格拉夫，保罗·弗鲁恩霍夫
波兰	创业与经济发展研究所，管理学院	帕韦尔·齐斯
葡萄牙	Tecninvest 研究与咨询公司	安东尼奥·科英布拉
西班牙	Ikei 研究与咨询	杰西卡·杜兰
英国	金士顿大学小型企业研究中心	伊娃·卡斯珀罗娃

致　谢

  本书的翻译得到了北京市委党校李兵教授的大力支持和帮助，翻译过程中，闫萍副教授和王雪梅副教授提供了中肯的意见和建议，校委委员袁吉富教授、科研处处长鄂振辉教授和林婧老师亦给予了很大的帮助，在此一并表示衷心的感谢！

  感谢本书编辑张潜博士的细致工作。

  最后，特别感谢欧洲基金（www. eurofound. europa. eu）Jan Vandamme 先生的大力支持。

汪　消

Abstract

This book examines recruitment and retention measures in community-based care and support services for adults with disabilities and health problems. It focuses on 10 EU Member States: Austria, Bulgaria, Denmark, France, Germany, the Netherlands, Poland, Portugal, Spain and the United Kingdom. It examines 30 case studies from these countries, analysing initiatives that were successful either in creating more jobs in the provision of health and social care for adults in the community or in improving the quality of jobs, with the aim of both attracting new recruits and retaining existing staff.

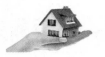

Policy context

Population ageing is generating a need and a demand for more and better jobs in long-term care. An accessible and high-quality system of health and social care provision is essential for European societies and economies. The health and social care sector is growing in nearly all EU Member States, providing opportunities for an ever greater number of jobs. This is a sector with increasing demands for quality and skills to support people with multiple chronic conditions. There are barriers to job creation in this sector, however, including a shortage of recruits, budgetary constraints and demanding working conditions. To overcome these problems and to support the creation of a strong workforce in the sector and its ongoing growth, a variety of strategies are required. Such strategies can be sustainable, however, only if workers find it worthwhile to stay in the sector, and this means that policies designed to solve labour shortages in the care sector must also ensure that they are satisfied with their working conditions and wages.

Key findings

(1) The balance of community-based versus institutional care

for adults with disabilities varies across countries. Overall, there is an increasing trend towards more community-based care. The momentum towards home care appears to be driven by lower costs, policies promoting the greater independence of people with disabilities, the preferences of clients and the potential of assisted-living technology.

(2) It is difficult to determine the size of the workforce in community-based care for the elderly and disabled. Data are available only for Austria (20,100 jobs), France (393,000 jobs), the Netherlands (132,200 jobs), Spain (115,900 jobs) and the UK (960,000 jobs).

(3) Data available for three of the study countries show rising numbers of home-care workers: on average, in Austria by 740 yearly, in France by 19,800 yearly and in the UK by 28,000 yearly. Most likely, this rising trend also applies in other countries. The rising trend is expected to continue in the coming years.

(4) Generally, the labour market for community-based care is characterized by shortages, especially at higher qualification levels. These have been mitigated temporarily by the economic crisis. In the long term, increasing shortages are to be expected, especially for better-qualified personnel. Europe is in the midst of an economic crisis that is leading to cutbacks in care services and more emphasis on the financial argument for community-based care over institutional

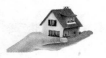

care. High unemployment rates are making the sector more attractive to work in, while the increasing emphasis on labour market measures may succeed in boosting recruitment.

Labour market strategies

Four labour market strategies have been identified to improve recruitment and retention in the sector: (1) targeting labour reserves in order to attract new employees to the sector, including the recruitment of unemployed people and groups such as immigrants and labour migrants; (2) promoting and facilitating the education of potential employees-by, for example, creating spe-cific learning paths, developing campaigns to encourage young people to choose a career in the sector and improving the relationship between this labour market and educational institutions; (3) improving the working conditions of current employees in order to optimise their potential and retain them in the sector-for instance, by introducing training programmes, professionalising the sector and providing more career opportunities for existing employees; (4) improving the operational management and labour productivity of organisations, for example through the use of new technologies and direct payments, or distributing tasks more effectively among staff.

Policy pointers

（1）Recruitment programmes in community-based care services can provide job opportunities for people in the migrant population, the long-term unemployed and adults who themselves have disabilities. Some migrants may already have experience in the informal care sector. Reaching each of these groups needs a targeted approach.

（2）Campaigns to encourage young people to consider a career in the care sector are more successful if targeted at specific groups. Much remains to be done to persuade boys especially that care work is a valid career choice.

（3）The content and organisation of social care education has to be attractive to students, with an emphasis on practical work and, if possible, traineeships in their own neighbourhood.

（4）For people already working in the sector, human resource and general management have to be professional. Standards in the care sector can be improved through practice-oriented training and retraining schemes for workers. Training is more successful if it is close to home, as much as possible free of charge and run during working hours; small class sizes are also recommended.

（5）Assistive technology offers much potential in this field. Workers need to be trained in the use of this technology. It is also

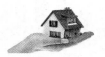

important to gain acceptance of the technology among clients and service providers.

(6) Sustainability deserves particular attention, especially in the case of subsidised projects. This means that projects subsidised from public funds need secure finances, activities need to be coordinated effectively and one body or organisation needs to take on the lead role.

(7) The transfer of successful initiatives to other regions, countries or sectors demands a well-thought-out strategy to embed the successful innovations in regular activities and policies. This may include using the EU funding for transnational partnerships.

(8) Political willingness to address the labour market problems in home care and community-based care is an important prerequisite for successful, sustainable and transferable measures. At the moment, there is a gap between policies and political commitment. Legislation exists but sustained political support is needed to further develop the labour market for home care.

(9) Political support is essential to continue the structural funding of recruitment and retention measures by the EU and its Member States.

(10) Data gathering and use of statistics could be substantially improved to develop, monitor, evaluate and adapt the relevant labour market policies of national and European authorities.

Contents

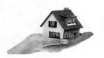 More and Better Jobs in Home-care Services

Introduction

1. Policy background

In February 2013, the European Commission in its Social Investment Package called on Member States to prioritise social investment and to modernise their welfare states in response to the significant challenges they face. These challenges include high levels of financial distress, increasing poverty and social exclusion, and record unemployment, especially among young people. These are compounded by the challenge posed by an ageing society and smaller working age populations, which tests the sustainability and adequacy of national social systems[1].

---

[1] European Commission (2013), Social Investment: Commission Urges Member States to Focus on Growth and Social Cohesion, press release, 20 February.

The Social Investment Package directs specific attention to long-term care in the Commission staff working document Long-term care in ageing societies—Challenges and policy options[1]. This document sets out how to reduce the need for long-term care through prevention, rehabilitation and the creation of more age-friendly environments, and by developing more efficient ways of delivering care.

A functioning and high-quality system of health and social care provision is essential for European societies and economies. Ill-health can lead to social exclusion and create barriers to participation in society. At the same, the health and social care sector is growing quickly, providing an ever greater number of " white job " opportunities[2]. As population ageing increases demand for high-quality care, there is yet more potential for employment growth in the sector. However, in its 2012 communication "Towards a job-rich recovery", the European Commission identified a number of barriers to job creation specifically in this sector[3]. These include: (1) the

---

[1] European Commission (2013), Long-term Care in Ageing Societies—Challenges and Policy Options, SWD(2013) 41 final, Brussels.

[2] When introducing the priorities of the current European Commission, President Barroso emphasised the fundamental need to create jobs and highlighted the opportunities for Europe of both "green jobs" (in sectors related to the environment and management of climate change) and "white jobs" (in health and social services).

[3] European Commission (2012), Towards a Job-rich Recovery, COM (2012) 173 final, Brussels.

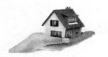

shortage of new recruits to replace those who are retiring; (2) the emergence of new healthcare patterns to tackle multiple chronic conditions; (3) budgetary constraints; (4) demanding working conditions with little compensation.

To overcome these problems and to support the creation of a strong and growing workforce in the sector, countries are already taking different measures to improve the situation. Other countries can learn from these.

2. Aim of the book

The main aim of the book is to examine job creation (including recruitment and retention) in the care sector. In particular it examines home and community-based care and support services for adults with physical or intellectual disabilities or chronic physical or mental health problems. It describes the current situation in selected Member States and highlights those measures that have proved successful in developing both the numbers and quality of the care workforce.

To achieve this main aim, the following specific objectives were set: (1) to identify 10 Member States where initiatives have been established to increase the number and quality of home-care workers or to decrease turnover rates of staff, and where policies and legislation are in place to promote the growth of the workforce of carers; (2) to describe the current labour market in home care and community-based care in the selected countries; (3) to document how and with what success the different recruitment and retention measures have been implemented in the selected countries.

3. Scope

At the centre of this book are jobs in home care and community-based care for disabled adults. Community-based care is defined as health and social care that is provided to people to enable them to live in a community[①]. It contrasts with institutional care, which is defined as care provided in residential institutions. Some sources distinguish between home care (instead of community-based care) and institutional care[②]. However, there are countries in which the term " home care " has a narrower meaning. Therefore the term

---

① There is overlap between community-based care and personal and household services (PHS). PHS are defined as a broad range of activities that contribute to the well-being of families and individuals at home: childcare, long-term care for the elderly and for people with disabilities, remedial classes, home repairs, gardening, ICT support and welfare work. See European Commission (2012), Commission Staff Working Document on Exploiting the Employment Potential of the Personal and Household Services, SWD(2012) 95 final, Strasbourg.

② See, for instance,Rodrigues, R. , Huber, M. and Lamura, G. (eds.) (2012), Facts and Figures on Healthy Ageing and Long-term Care, European Centre for Social Welfare Policy and Research, Vienna. Here home care is defined as care provided at home by professionals after a formal needs assessment. "Care" means domestic aid services, personal care, and supportive, technical and rehabilitative nursing.

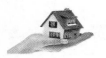

"community-based care" is used in preference, while at the same time the people involved are called "home-care workers", which better describes their activities than the term "community-based care workers".

In this book, home-care workers are defined as health and social care workers who: (1) provide health and social care services to a specific target group (adults with a physical or intellectual disability, or with chronic physical or mental health problems, particularly people below retirement age); (2) provide care of a specific type (long-term care); (3) work in a specific setting (community-based care as opposed to institutional care); (4) work in a formal (waged) context (as opposed to informal, non-waged care).

This definition shows that the discussion does not address one specific occupation or profession. A profession often defines itself by a specific professional identity, a professional history or self-organisation. An occupation is mostly defined by the qualifications that someone needs to have acquired to be able to enter that sector's labour market and continue practising in the occupation. Definitions of professions and occupations can, however, differ considerably across different countries[1].

---

① Cedefop (European Centre for the Development of Vocational Training) (2012), The Role of Qualifications in Governing Occupations and Professions, Cedefop, Thessaloniki.

This book, therefore, concentrates on the type and objectives of the activities carried out in the labour market as described above. Based on these activities, this book focuses on a number of occupational groups roughly corresponding to NACE code 88. 10 (social work activities without accommodation for the elderly and disabled), including home carers, social care workers, social workers, activity workers[1], community nurses and other professions, such as therapists. Certain occupational groups in primary healthcare, such as family doctors and dentists, are excluded.

4. Selection of Member States

This book studies 10 Member States in depth, the selection of which was based on the following criteria: (1) geographical location: countries from all four regions of Europe (north, east, south and west); (2) accession group: countries from different accession groups, distinguishing between the 15 Member States prior to the 2004 enlargement, the 2004 accession countries and the 2007 accession countries; (3) degree of deinstitutionalisation: countries with low rates of home care and community-based care and countries

---

[1] Staff supporting people in community activities or activities aimed to reintegrate people into employment.

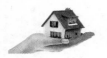

with high rates; (4) existence of relevant policies, legislation and initiatives: countries for which it has been shown that there are shortages of home-care workers and that there are relevant policies, laws and initiatives to increase recruitment.

On the basis of these indicators, a provisional selection was made. To get a first impression of the variety of issues, policy approaches and potentially interesting cases for deeper study, the experts in the countries concerned carried out some brief desk-based research. They looked at the general topic and developments in the field, while also identifying some examples of initiatives aimed at resolving the issues.

While the characteristics of the sector are similar across the countries, the economic and policy context of a country (for instance, in terms of general policies, legislation, level of centralisation, formal versus informal care and funding structure) determines how these issues are discussed and what the responses are in terms of policies, instruments and initiatives.

The following final selection of Member States was made: Austria, Bulgaria, Denmark, France, Germany, the Netherlands, Poland, Portugal, Spain and the United Kingdom.

5. Research activities

Three models were used to construct a methodological approach. (1) The labour market model maps the current and expected situation in demand and supply and problems relating to discrepancies between demand and supply in the labour market. (2) The PESTLE analysis describes the political, economic, social, technological, legal and environmental factors influencing the labour market. (3) The solutions model classifies measures to resolve the problems in the labour market.

These three models, which are described in detail in Annex 1, formed the basis for formulating specific research questions, the collection and analysis of data and the reporting.

The book started with desk-based research on relevant EU policies and EU statistics.

Next, in each of the 10 selected countries, national experts from the European Network for Social and Economic Research (ENSR) gathered relevant country information (see Annex 2 for the names and organisations of the experts). By using a fixed template it was possible to collect country information in a structured manner.

The national experts produced similar types of country reports that were readily comparable and from which conclusions could be

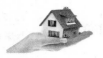

drawn. Globally, the themes were: (1) the context in which policies and initiatives are developed and the problems they aim to address; (2) political and legal frameworks; (3) the structural framework and funding structure; (4) types of programmes deployed for recruitment and retention of employees.

In addition, the national experts carried out 30 case studies on successful initiatives in the field of home-care job creation and retention. Model cases were selected to represent of the following four strategies to resolve problems with the labour market in this sector: (1) targeting labour reserves; (2) stimulating and facilitating education for potential employees; (3) improving the circumstances of current employees; (4) improving the operational management and labour productivity of organisations.

The most important selection criteria were that the approaches had to be both innovative and practical. An innovative and practical approach was defined as any project, policy or solution that: (1) attempts to increase the number or quality of workers or decrease the turnover rates of staff; (2) aims specifically at workers delivering community care services for adults with physical or intellectual disabilities or chronic physical or mental health problems; (3) addresses specific qualitative and quantitative discrepancies and lack of transparency in the labour market of care workers; (4) addresses one or more of the four strategies to combat labour market discrepancies; (5) has a clear and dynamic vision and approach; (6) has specified the conditions under which the approach operates; (7) follows and carefully registers processes and procedures; (8) has proven to be successful, having been evaluated at least once and shown visible effects (in terms of target groups reached, follow-ups, intrinsic and extrinsic effects).

In addition to being innovative and practical, the initiatives also had to be substantial in outreach, staff and funding. Within each strategy, a variety of types of measure were selected. The resulting mixture of selected cases is assumed to represent high-quality and transferable examples of initiatives and approaches to recruiting and retaining staff, beneficial for policymakers in all EU Member States.

Globally, each case study comprised five parts. (1) Problem definition: What specific labour market problem does the initiative address? (2) Approach: What approach has been used to address the problem? What are the core elements of the approach? (3)Contextual factors: What conditions have influenced the good practice identified? What fac-tors improved the success of the initiative? (4) Results: What have been the results of the initiative? How many jobs have been created? Has the problem been solved? (5) Lessons learnt: What can the organisations directly involved and others learn from this particular initiative? What are the main success and failure factors? How sustainable is the

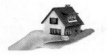

initiative? To what extent is the approach transferable to other situations?

On the basis of an analysis of the 30 case studies, it was possible to draw conclusions about success and potential failure factors, to determine the sustainability and transferability of recruitment and retention measures, and to formulate policy pointers for job-creation policies.

6. Book structure

Chapter One describes the EU policy context and presents statistics on expenditure in the health and social care sector in Europe, the recipients of care, and employment in the sector. Chapter Two describes the characteristics of this labour market and the contextual factors influencing it. Chapter Three presents an overview of the 30 case studies of good practice in recruitment and retention in the sector, classifying them on the basis of the labour market strategy they exemplify. Chapter Four provides a summary of the outcomes of the initiatives and the impact they have had on employment. Chapter Five discusses the factors associated with success and failure in the initiatives. Chapter Six draws a number of conclusions from the study and offers a list of policy pointers.

The annexes at the end of the book comprise the analytical

framework of the study and an overview of the national experts involved in this research project. The 10 countries' studies including the case studies are set out in separate books.

Chapter One: European Policies and Statistics on Health and Social Care

This chapter begins with an outline of relevant EU policies concerning the health and social care sector. The recent Social Investment Package, which urges Member States to prioritise social investment and to modernise their welfare states, is especially relevant. The discussion summarises the policies that address future EU health workforce needs, focusing on five themes: workforce planning, anticipation of skills requirements, training and mobility, recruitment and retention, and EU funding. The chapter then presents EU statistics related to the labour market in care and support services for adults with disabilities or health problems.

1. EU policies

(1) Europe 2020

Europe 2020 is a 10-year strategy proposed by the European Commission on 3 March 2010 for the advancement of the economy of the European Union. The strategy aims to achieve "smart, sustainable, inclusive growth" with greater coordination of national and European policy[1].

A report by the Social Protection Committee in 2011 analysing the social dimension of the Europe 2020 strategy delivered 10 key messages. One of the key messages was to increase the effectiveness, sustainability and responsiveness of healthcare and long-term care[2].

The EU promotes the coordination of national long-term care policies through the open method of coordination[3], with a particular focus on access, quality and sustainability. For this book, the most relevant objectives in these three areas are: (1) enhancing the provision of long-term care services (a mix of home, community and

---

① European Commission (2010), Europe 2020: A Strategy for Smart, Sustainable and Inclusive Growth, COM(2010) 2020 final, Brussels.

② European Commission (2011), The Social Dimension of the Europe 2020 Strategy: A Report of the Social Protection Committee, Publications Office of the European Union, Luxembourg.

③ The open method of coordination (OMC) is a framework for cooperation between the Member States. The outcomes of the OMC have a potentially binding character but are actually "soft law"—they depend upon peer pressure.

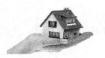

institutional services) to all layers of the population; (2) reducing geographical differences in availability and quality of care; (3) prioritising tailor-made care and support services to ensure that people live in their home for as long as possible; and, where these services are not available, their promotion via a parallel adaptation of the institutional care setting; (4) creating quality assurance measures; (5) placing emphasis on health promotion at all ages including old age, disease prevention and rehabilitation policies; (6) ensuring sufficient human resources through formal staff training, motivation and working conditions.

Another important goal to address the expected shortage of labour in the health and care sector is "to facilitate and promote intra-EU labour mobility and better match labour supply and demand with appropriate financial support from the structural funds"[1]. The EU has also developed several concrete actions to improve the long-term care sector.

(2) Employment Package

The Employment Package (launched in April 2012) is a set of policy documents that examines how EU employment policies

---

[1] European Commission (2010), Europe 2020: A Strategy for Smart, Sustainable and Inclusive Growth, COM(2010) 2020 final, Brussels, p. 18.

intersect with a number of other policy areas in support of smart, sustainable and inclusive growth[①]. It identifies the areas that offer the greatest job potential in the EU and the most effective ways for EU countries to create more jobs.

As the health and social care sector has high employment potential, the Employment Package pays special attention to white jobs and includes an action plan for the EU health workforce. This plan sets out actions to foster European cooperation and share good practice to help improve health workforce planning and forecasting, to anticipate future skills needs and to improve the recruitment and retention of health professionals, while mitigating the negative effects of migration on health systems.

As part of the Employment Package, the Commission also published a staff working document on exploiting the potential of personal and household services[②]. This package aims to identify strategies for dealing with the following: (1) better work-life balance, achieved through increased transfer of daily tasks done in the home to service providers, as well as child and elderly care; (2) job creation for the relatively low-skilled, particularly in

---

① European Commission (2012), Towards a Job-rich Recovery, COM (2012) 173 final, Brussels.

② European Commission (2012), Commission Staff Working Document on Exploiting the Employment Potential of the Personal and Household Services, SWD(2012) 95 final, Strasbourg.

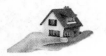

housework services; (3) improvement in the quality of care.

In consultation with the stakeholders (including national authorities, social partners and service users and suppliers), these strategies will be further developed.

(3) Social Investment Package

The 2013 Social Investment Package sets out the EU policy framework and concrete actions to be taken by Member States and the Commission so that social protection systems are more efficient and effective, with guidance on the use of EU funds to support reforms.

An important component of the Social Investment Package is the Commission staff working document Long-term Care in Ageing Societies—Challenges and Policy Options[①]. It argues that Europe needs to prepare for a tripling of the number of people in the age group most likely to need long-term care (people aged 80 years and over) by 2060. The current modes of responding to older people's long-term care needs are not sustainable in view of this major demographic shift. The document highlights ways of responding to this challenge by reducing the need for long-term care through

---

① European Commission (2013), Long-term Care in Ageing Societies—Challenges and Policy Options, SWD(2013) 41 final, Brussels.

prevention of illness, rehabilitation and the creation of more age-friendly environments, and by developing more efficient ways of delivering care.

The EU can play a major role in promoting innovation and social investment in this area by developing new ways of closing the gap between long-term care needs and provision through, for example, the European Innovation Partnership on Active and Healthy Ageing and the Ambient Assisted Living Programme. The EU can also use the structural funds to boost investment in age-friendly environments and better-qualified professional carers.

Progress towards financially sustainable and socially adequate social protection against long-term care risks will continue to be monitored by the EU's Economic Policy and Social Protection Committees. This will be decisive for achieving a number of goals set in the context of the Europe 2020 strategy—sound public finances in ageing societies, a high level of employment and the reduction of poverty.

The Commission document on long-term care recommends that Member States give particular attention to strategies oriented towards social investment that combine preventive measures of healthy and active ageing with productivity drives in care delivery and measures to increase the ability of older men and women to continue independent living even as they become frail or develop disabilities.

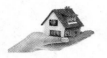

Moreover, as increasing priority is given to the quality of public expenditure in EU policy guidance through country-specific policy pointers, these should also focus on improving the effectiveness of spending in this area, so that adequate social protection against long-term care risks can be ensured even at the height of population ageing.

2. Policy actions

The Member States recognise the challenges of the health and social care sector and therefore, at an EPSCO (Employment, Social Policy, Health and Consumer Affairs Council) meeting in December 2010, invited the Commission to assist Member States in tackling long-term issues around the health workforce. In the section below, several of the actions and measures that the EU has developed in recent years are discussed. These actions are grouped around the five key issues of workforce planning, skills anticipation, training and labour mobility, recruitment and retention practices, and funding through the EU structural funds.

(1) Workforce planning

According to the Commission, health workforce planning is one of the biggest challenges facing Europe today. At the moment, the lack of comparable statistics makes forecasts unreliable. As a consequence, an EU Joint Action on Health Workforce Planning and Forecasting (2013 – 2015) has been put in place. In a feasibility study to identify actions that could be carried out at EU level to support workforce planning, the Commission indicated that the EU could support the creation of common definitions, indicators, tools and methodologies, and will work closely with data collectors such as Eurostat, the OECD and the World Health Organization[①]. A coordinating role has been suggested for the European Observatory on Health Workforce Planning (created after the 2008 Green Paper on the health workforce). The action programme aims to provide comparable statistics and new, reliable forecasting models. The forecasts will take a central position in formulating policy interventions in education, training, working conditions and recruitment of healthcare workers.

(2) Skills anticipation

A second challenge is identifying the skills that will be necessary for long-term care workers. Shifting care from institutions to people's homes, the use of new technologies and the use of

① Matrix Insight (2012), EU Level Collaboration on Forecasting Health Workforce Needs, Workforce Planning and Health Workforce Trends—A Feasibility Study, European Commission Executive Agency for Health and Consumers, Luxembourg.

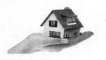

different diagnostic techniques all influence the skills that will be relevant in the future. The EU is developing several projects to map skills and competences in the healthcare sector: it is investigating the feasibility of a European Sector Council on Employment and Skills for the Nursing and Care Workforce, and a pilot network of healthcare assistants is being put into place. These two projects will contribute to the EU Skills Panorama, which will provide an overview of emerging skills needs and will contain a common multilingual classification of occupations and skills. A skills forecast from Cedefop (the European Centre for the Development of Vocational Training) will be another building block of this panorama.

(3) Training and labour mobility

The third challenge focuses on providing people with the correct training to prevent a mismatch between job requirements and education. In August 2012, a call for proposals to create a pilot Sector Skills Alliance for the healthcare sector closed. This alliance brings together educational providers, sector experts (such as sector federations) and public and private education authorities to create new curricula and training methods to provide students with skills demanded by the labour market. Erasmus for All 2012 – 2014 is an EU funding programme to increase cross-border education that also applies to healthcare workers. Both policies can be seen in the light of the Lifelong Learning Programme and the commitment to continuous professional development. The Commission states in a directive on professional qualifications that Member States need to mutually recognise professional qualifications. The goal is to increase the motivation and professional competences of healthcare workers and to increase cross-border labour mobility. Mobility and migration are deemed important because labour market shortages tend to be geographically dispersed.

(4) Recruitment and retention practices

European social dialogue in the hospital and healthcare sector plays an important role in sharing knowledge about recruitment and retention practices. In this dialogue the European Federation of Public Service Unions (EPSU) and the European Hospital and Healthcare Employers' Association (HOSPEEM) develop guidelines, standards and best practices. This led, for example, to a framework of actions on recruitment and retention in 2010 and a code of conduct for cross-border recruitment.

(5) Funding through the EU structural funds

The EU is directly involved in improving the health and care sector by allocating funding through the EU structural funds. The

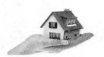

Commission states in its 2012 action plan for the EU health workforce that "Member states are urged to maximise the use of European funding instruments to support actions to tackle workforce shortages and to boost job creation in the healthcare sector"①.

The two most relevant funds are the European Social Fund (ESF) and the European Regional Development Fund (ERDF). The ERDF can stimulate infrastructural and more technical elements of the care sectors (for instance, building a community-based care centre) and the ESF focuses primarily on creating better-skilled personnel and promoting social inclusion. In the recently adopted regulation of the ESF 2014 – 2020, there is a stronger focus on employment, labour mobility and lifelong learning. This could mean that more funds will be allocated to job creation and retention in the care sector.

The Ad Hoc Expert Group on the Transition from Institutional to Community-based Care advocates increasing investment in community-based care. In a 2012 communication on healthy ageing, the Commission stresses the priority "to a shift from institutional care to community-based care, while enhancing independent living"②, a

---

① European Commission (2012), Commission Staff Working Document on an Action Plan for the EU Health Workforce, SWD(2012) 93 final, Strasbourg, p. 12.

② European Commission (2012), Taking Forward the Strategic Implementation Plan of the European Innovation Partnership on Active and Healthy Ageing, COM(2012) 83 final, Brussels, p. 11.

point it also makes in its disability strategy.

In summary, the EU has no mandate to enforce rules in the area of health and social care and employment. However, it has shown a strong commitment to improving the accessibility, sustainability and quality of the health and care sector. Although this is done primarily by coordination and goal-setting, the EU's targets have been translated recently into concrete pilot projects that investigate how the health and social care sector as a whole (and, in particular, long-term care for an ageing population) can be supported by a thriving, motivated and professionally qualified workforce. Moreover, the EU welcomes funding proposals to improve the health and social care sector.

3. EU statistics

There are numerous EU-wide statistics on the health and social care services sector. These statistics are, however, limited in two ways. Many statistics do not distinguish between institutional and home or community-based care. Secondly, most long-term care statistics do not differentiate between services for the various age groups (children, adults under retirement age and older people above retirement age). The statistics on expenditure, recipients and employment presented in this section should therefore be interpreted

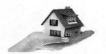

with these limitations in mind[1].

(1) Expenditure

According to the 2012 ageing report, in 2012, 1.8% of GDP was spent on long-term care in the EU27[2]. It notes that long-term care spending varies considerably across EU countries: the Netherlands spends 3.8% of its GDP on long-term care, Austria 1.2% and Estonia only 0.2%. Although most people receive care in home-based settings, this type of care reflects only between 30% and 50% of spending, which would mean that home-based care represents approximately 0.6% to 0.9% of the EU27's GDP[3]. It should also be noted that in relation to this specific type of care, there are large differences between countries (See Figure 1).

---

① Sources dealing with the limitations associated with statistics on the health and social care services include Huber, M. (2007), Monitoring Long-term Care in Europe: Background Paper on Care Indicators, European Centre for Social Welfare Policy and Research, Vienna, and European Commission (2006), The Impact of Ageing on Public Expenditure: Projections for the EU25 Member States on Pensions, Health Care, Long-term Care, Education and Unemployment Transfers (2004 – 2050), Special Report No. 1/2006, Economic Policy Committee and the Directorate-General of Economic and Financial Affairs, Brussels. See also the SHARE (Survey of Health, Ageing and Retirement in Europe) study, 2012, at http://www.share-project.org/.

② European Commission (2012), The 2012 Ageing Report: Economic and Budgetary Projections for the 27 EU Member States (2010 – 2060), European Commission, Brussels.

③ Rodrigues, R., Huber, M. and Lamura, G. (eds.) (2012), Facts and Figures on Healthy Ageing and Long-term Care, European Centre for Social Welfare Policy and Research, Vienna.

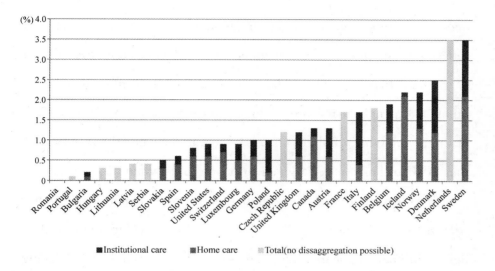

Figure 1   Public expenditure on long-term care (as a percentage of GDP) in different care settings in Europe and North America, 2009 or most recent year

Note: "Total" represent data for which no reliable information by care setting is available. The figure does not take into account private spending on care, which explains the somewhat unexpected order of countries (for example, the US being among the low-spending countries).

Source: Rodrigues, R., Huber, M. and Lamura, G. (eds.) (2012), Facts and Figures on Healthy Ageing and Long-term Care, European Centre for Social Welfare Policy and Research, Vienna.

(2) Recipients of long-term care

On average 2. 3% of the population used formal long-term care services across OECD countries in 2008. About one-fifth of recipients are aged 64 or younger. It is estimated that only 1% of those under 65 have some kind of long-term care. More than half of long-term care is provided in the home or in community-based care settings,

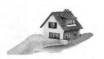

and this proportion is on average higher for recipients below retirement age than above, as stated in the 2011 reports: *Health at a glance* and *Help wanted?*[1]. There are large country differences in the number of people using formal long-term care services, from 0.2% of the population in Poland to 5.1% in Austria. The OECD estimates that 80% of home care is given to people older than 65.

It is expected that the number of people in home-based care will increase by 130% by 2050, since there is a clear trend towards deinstitutionalising care, an increase in demand caused by ageing and a reduction in the availability of informal carers[2]. The trend towards community-based care is also reflected in the fact that the vast majority of respondents to the 2007 special Eurobarometer on health and long-term care stated that they would prefer community-based care rather than institutional care[3]. Community-based care is thus of great relevance for adults below retirement age who receive long-term care, even though this group is small in absolute numbers.

---

[1]   OECD (2011), Health at a Glance 2011-OECD Indicators, OECD Publishing, Paris. OECD (2011), Help Wanted? Providing and Paying for Long-term Care, OECD Publishing, Paris.

[2]   European Commission (2006), The Impact of Ageing on Public Expenditure: Projections for the EU25 Member States on Pensions, Health Care, Long-term Care, Education and Unemployment Transfers (2004 – 2050), Special Report No. 1/2006, Economic Policy Committee and the Directorate-General of Economic and Financial Affairs, Brussels.

[3]   European Commission (2007), Health and Long-term Care in the European Union, Special Eurobarometer 283, European Commission, Brussels.

(3) Labour demand

The OECD estimates that long-term care is the fastest-growing division within the health and social care sector[1]. It is expected that the number of people working in long-term care will double by 2050. This growth is driven by the increasing number of elderly people demanding care and by a reduction of available informal carers[2]. Other drivers for this growing demand include changing patterns of disease and changing attitudes and expectations concerning care and quality of life. Regrettably, there are no statistics that break down the long-term workforce structure by different types of care. A good approximation might be that used by the OECD for the recipients of long-term care, suggesting that approximately 80% of workers in the sector are involved in care for the elderly.

Home-care and community-based care services are one way of providing care and support for older people and for those with disabilities in a financially sustainable manner. These kinds of services are already prevalent across the EU. According to data for 2010 from Eurostat, personal services-partly overlapping with

---

① OECD (2011), Help Wanted? Providing and Paying for Long-term Care, OECD Publishing, Paris.

② European Commission (2012), The 2012 Ageing Report: Economic and Budgetary Projections for the 27 EU Member States (2010 – 2060), European Commission, Brussels.

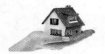

home care services-represented 5.4 million jobs in the EU, a number that will increase in the future to respond to growing demand[①].

① Andor, L. (2011), We Care, How can the EU Care?, Conference Presentation, Social Platform's Annual Conference on Care, 9 December, Brussels.

Chapter Two : Labour Market Context

This chapter describes the context in which recruitment and retention measures in care and support services for adults with disabilities or health problems are developed and implemented. It is based on a number of recent European publications and on information from the 10 countries that the national experts have reported on for this book. Topics cover the proportion of home care in total care, the characteristics of this labour market and the contextual factors influencing the labour market for jobs in care and support services.

1. Home care versus institutional care

The proportion of long-term home care versus institutional care

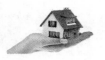

for adults with disabilities varies from country to country. Figure 2 illustrates this for people aged 65 years and over (as a rule, the proportion of care and support services for disabled people under 65

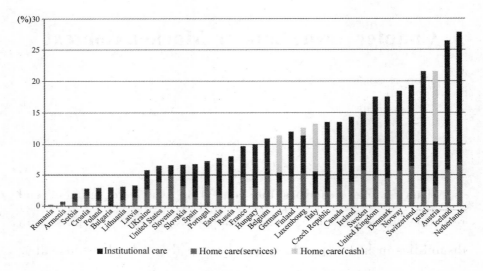

Figure 2   Percentage of people aged 65 and older receiving institutional care, state-provided home care or cash for the purchase of care services, 2009 or most recent year

Notes: Data for Belgium and Austria are for people aged 60 + ; France, for people aged 60 + for home care. Some of the national sources refer to age groups that may not coincide with the 65 + cut-off. "Home care (services)" includes those taking a combination of cash and state-provided services. Estimates for Italy's "Home care(cash)" category are a conservative approximation so as to avoid double-counting. Disaggregated data for Luxembourg and Germany are extrapolated from total beneficiaries. Private spending on care is not taken into account, and there has been no correction for the demographic factor that some countries have older populations than others.

Source: Rodrigues, R. , Huber, M. and Lamura, G. (eds.) (2012), Facts and Figures on Healthy Ageing and Long-term Care, European Centre for Social Welfare Policy and Research, Vienna.

is smaller than that for people aged 65 and older).

Despite the differences between countries, the analysis of the country studies shows a clear overall preference for non-institutional over institutional care. In general, the social and political climate in European countries is favourable to care at home.

One reason for providing more non-institutionalised care is the reduction of costs, motivated by the rising demand and the economic crisis. In general, governments see home care and community-based care as less expensive than institutionalised care. There are no costs for housing or buildings, overheads are lower, and there are more incentives for neighbours and family to assist in care. However, there are the costs associated with travelling to the clients, although these may be mitigated by the use of information and communication technologies (ICTs) and better organisation of home care at the district level.

Another reason for increasing the level of home care by governments is to enable patients to live and act independently in their own environment for as long as possible. Clients usually prefer home care to institutionalised care, as the recent Home Care across Europe report shows[1]. The one exception is Slovenia, where

---

① Genet, N., Boerma, W., Kroneman, M., Hutchinson, A., and Saltman, R. B. (eds.) (2012), Home Care across Europe: Current Structure and Future Challenges, Observatory Studies No. 27, World Health Organization, Copenhagen.

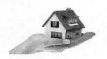

More and Better Jobs in Home-care Services

institutionalised care is preferred for dependent elderly people. The reason for these differing preferences is unknown, and further research may be able to clarify the special situation in Slovenia.

Additionally, as a result of developments in assisted-living technology, care at home has become more feasible.

2. Labour market characteristics

In this book, the labour market model in Annex 1 was used to map the discrepancies between demand and supply in the labour market in home care and community-based care. This section first describes—as far as is possible with the available data—the size of the labour market (demand side). Then it elaborates on the discrepancies between demand and supply in the labour market.

(1) Extent of employment in care

The information available for home and community-based care as a whole is scattered and only partially comparable. For some countries included in this study, data on employment in NACE code 88. 10 (social work activities without accommodation for the elderly and disabled) was available. In addition to NACE 88. 10 figures, some national experts were able to give employment figures on a higher aggregation level. Table 1 presents a summary of available data.

Table 1　**Estimated number of employees in care and support services for adults with disabilities**

Country	Employment in NACE 88.10	Other relevant employment figures
Austria	In 2012, 20,095 employed people (compared with 17,140 in 2008); average yearly growth of +740	Besides professionals, on average 9,300 people are carrying out compulsory civilian services (partly in social care)
Bulgaria	No information available on NACE 88.10	In 2011, the number of employees in human health and social work activities as a whole was 153,500, compared with 122,513 in 2006. In 2011, 28,075 people were employed in residential care and social work activities (compared with 27,990 in 2009)
Denmark	No information available on NACE 88.10	In 2011, the number of health and social care workers and assistants[a] in total was 122,918, compared with 119,644 in 2008
France	In 2010, 393,700 employees, of which 261,400 were in community support work (NACE 88.10A) and 122,100 in employment support work (NACE 88.10C). Numbers are increasing: compared to 2008, +16% in community support work (NACE 88.10A) and +3% in employment support work (NACE 88.10C); average yearly growth NACE 88.10A and 88.10C combined: +19,800	The number of hours worked in home-care services represents 429,000 full-time equivalent jobs on the basis of a 35-hour week (legal duration of working week in France). Most of these hours correspond to home-help hours and are classified under NACE 97.00 "Activities of households as employers of domestic personnel"
Germany	No information available on NACE 88.10	At the end of 2009, the total number of employees providing formal (waged) care on behalf of the Social Long-term Care Insurance Scheme was 890,283, of which 268,900 were active in the field of home care and community-based care

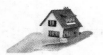 More and Better Jobs in Home-care Services

(contd.)

Country	Employment in NACE 88.10	Other relevant employment figures
Netherlands	In 2012, there were 2, 055 establishments with—according to the roughest estimate—132, 300 employed people[b]	In 2011, the number of jobs in the health and social care sector as a whole was 1,348,900. The branches of mental care, care for the handicapped, home-care services and welfare services accounted for respectively 88,000, 161,000, 193,000 and 72,000 jobs (in total 514,000 jobs)
Poland	No information available on NACE 88.10	In 2011, in total around 650,000 people were employed in professions related to health and social care[c] There are no detailed data on the number of people delivering long-term healthcare. In 2011 around 7,000 employees were working in the Social Assistance Centres delivering social care (general care services and specialist care services)[d]
Portugal	No information available on NACE 88.10	In 2010 there were about 6,100 private facilities or services providing social care (NACE 87 and 88, that is, residential care and social care respectively), both for-profit and not-for-profit, and employing about 114,900 people (of whom 61,800 were in NACE 87 and 53,100 in NACE 88). Around 113,200 people were employed in 2008 (of whom 59,200 were in NACE 87 and 54,000 in NACE 88)
Spain	In 2012 there were 2, 489 establishments with 115, 900 employees (compared with 2,348 establishments and 102, 300 employees in 2009)	

(contd.)

Country	Employment in NACE 88.10	Other relevant employment figures
UK	In 2009, there were 4,720 registered businesses (public, commercial and voluntary/ charitable) across the UK, with approximately 960,000 employees (3% increase on 2008 and 9% increase on 2005); average yearly growth based on 2008-2009 figures: +28,000	There were an estimated 1.85 million jobs in adult social care in England alone in 2011 (an increase of 4.5% on 2010), while the actual workforce in adult social care stood at 1.63 million. The split between residential and non-residential establishments is 48% and 52% respectively. Most jobs in social care (65%) are provided by independent employers, followed by direct-payment recipients (23%), local authorities (9%) and the NHS (4%)

Notes: [a] Occupations include nurse, physiotherapist, occupational therapist, teacher/educator, social educator, psychologist, social worker, social educator assistants, social and healthcare worker, social and healthcare/teaching assistant, social and health assistant.

[b] This is a rough estimate by the authors based on data from the Dutch Central Statistical Office on the number of establishments with employees in NACE 88.10 and the classification of those employees. Estimates are: lowest—18,900 employees; middle—39,585 employees; highest—132,270 employees.

[c] Numbers in occupations related to health and social care, according to the International Standard Classification of Occupations (ISCO-88): 513 personal care and related workers, 223 nursing and midwifery associate professionals, 323 nursing and midwifery associate professionals and 913 domestic and related helpers, cleaners and laundry workers.

[d] This shows only a part of the labour force delivering long-term social care services, as social care services at beneficiaries' homes are subcontracted by the municipality's Social Assistance Centres to private companies. Data on the number of employees of these companies are not collected.

Source: Information supplied by national experts.

Though incomplete and only partly comparable, the picture derived from the country reports is one of growing numbers of home-

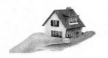

care workers in general, but also in the specific field of care for adults with disabilities.

The Home Care across Europe report confirms the lack of data in this field. Data on the number of home-care workers were not widely available for the purposes of this review[1].

(2) Discrepancies between labour demand and supply

Generally, the situation in the home-care labour market is not favourable. First of all, there are quantitative discrepancies. The Home Care across Europe report noted a general shortage of staff in several countries: Austria, Belgium, Bulgaria, Cyprus, Czech Republic, Finland, France, Greece, Lithuania, Portugal and Slovenia[2].

Secondly, there are qualitative discrepancies. In the same study, a number of countries—Bulgaria, Cyprus, Denmark, Estonia, France, Germany, Greece, Luxembourg and Norway— reported a lack of sufficiently qualified home care staff. For instance, Belgium and Bulgaria have too few home helps, while France, Greece, Lithuania and Slovenia have too few home-care professionals in general.

---

① Genet, N., Boerma, W., Kroneman, M., Hutchinson, A., and Saltman, R. B. (eds.) (2012), Home Care across Europe: Current Structure and Future Challenges, Observatory Studies No. 27, World Health Organization, Copenhagen.

② Ibid..

From the perspective of the care workers, there are qualitative discrepancies. In general, job quality (remuneration and other terms of employment, working conditions and working times) is less favourable than in other sectors: home care is a demanding job, some workers have more than one employer and work for two or more people on the same day, and working time can also be an issue. In some European countries, however, collective agreements by the social partners have led to the improvement of job quality.

The sector also has image problems, partly due to objective factors (terms of employment and working conditions) and partly due to subjective factors (negative perception and public sentiment). In general, image problems tend to be persistent and hard to combat.

In addition to this more general picture, some country-specific developments were reported by the national experts, as documented below.

Austria: While there is a rising demand for elderly-care workers, home helps and social workers, demand for disability-care workers in general remains constant. Nevertheless, job prospects in care for people with disabilities are very good for well-qualified personnel.

Bulgaria: Though no figures are available, there are signs that—as a result of the economic crisis—Bulgarian care workers

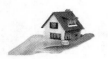

employed in countries such as Spain, Greece and Italy are returning to Bulgaria. This may temporarily alleviate the shortage of care workers in Bulgaria.

Denmark: As in most other countries, the community-based care and home-care workforce is comparatively old. Furthermore, a high turnover among social care and healthcare assistants compared to many other professions is reported. Attracting and retaining home-care workers appears to be especially difficult in the rural areas of Denmark.

France: The percentage of employers in the care sector expecting difficulties in recruiting increased from 61% in 2011 to 67% in 2012 (compared to 43% in 2012 for all sectors). These difficulties were mainly expected to be a lack of candidates (77%), their lack of skills, diplomas and motivation (67%), and the poor working conditions in the sector (45%).

Germany: The community-based care and home-care labour market has already been proved to be out of balance. In March 2012, there were only 3,268 registered unemployed care sector workers with adequate training per 10,000 vacant jobs. However, the number of unemployed people seeking a job in the care sector varies considerably across the regions. At present, the labour market suffers particularly from a shortage of skilled employees.

Netherlands: Due to the cost-reduction policies of the Dutch government, there is a labour surplus in welfare work, while there is a shortage of labour in healthcare.

Poland: Nurses still migrate to other EU Member States (especially in northern Europe) where the terms of employment and working conditions are better. This has increased labour shortages in the sector in Poland.

Portugal: In general, at the moment there is no shortage of care workers in Portugal, mainly as a result of the very high unemployment rate. This particularly applies to the higher-qualified segment of workers in the sector. At the moment, there are more than 100,000 unemployed workers with higher educational qualifications, many of them in fields relevant to the social sector. In some regions, however, there are some shortages of unqualified or poorly qualified workers.

Spain: The black economy appears to be a problem in the community-based care and home-care sector in Spain. In this irregular labour market, in which mainly poorly qualified women, especially migrants, are active, the terms of employment and working conditions are unfavourable. The irregular labour market seems to increase during crisis periods because non-professional services are cheaper. This is a significant obstacle to the professionalisation of the sector and the improvement of the terms of employment and working conditions for disadvantaged workers.

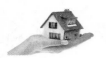

UK: Historically, social work and social care in the UK are characterised by labour shortages, a reliance on overtime work and temporary or inexperienced staff, poor management and high levels of bureaucracy, a lack of flexible working arrangements, the need to work anti-social hours and work of a stressful and demanding nature. Furthermore, many employers in this sector employ migrant workers from EU and non-EU countries.

(3) Expected developments

For the moment, labour shortages in the sector have been mitigated by the economic crisis, which has made work in the sector more popular. In the long term, the shortage of home-care workers is expected to increase, especially amongst higher-qualified workers. The supply of care workers cannot keep up with the rising demand for labour in the sector.

Information supplied by the national experts on expected developments in this labour market are documented here.

Austria: The demand for social care professionals who can, for instance, deliver care for the elderly or people with disabilities as well as offer life-coaching and social counselling will rise by 4,500 people, or 3.4% a year, until 2016. One cause of this is the approaching shift in the age structure of the population.

Until 2020, it is estimated that 6,400 additional full-time care workers will be needed in mobile services for elderly people, people with disabilities and other dependents. Chronic illnesses and mobility restrictions that result in many years of nursing or care needs will become more relevant than intensive medical treatments.

While there is a rising demand for elderly-care workers, home helps and social workers, demand for disability-care workers in general remains constant.

Bulgaria: In view of the increasing demand for community-based care and home care, an estimated employment growth of 500 to 1,000 people a year is expected.

Denmark: In the light of the global financial crisis, the overall problem of labour market shortages is considerably lower than in the recent past. However, in the long term, there will be shortages of home-care workers caused by, among other things, a growing elderly population and a shrinking labour force.

France: The general trend in the home-care sector is growth.

Germany: There is already a labour shortage in the German care sector. This is expected to increase as Germany's healthcare sector is expected to grow annually by at least 3%.

Netherlands: At the moment, the shortages in community-based healthcare are relatively small [mainly at qualification level 3 (intermediate vocational level) and for some specific professions], but in the coming years these shortages probably will increase,

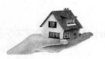

particularly at the higher-qualification levels. Due to the cost-reduction policies of the Dutch government, there is and will be a surplus of labour in welfare-related social care. The qualifications, skills and competences that employers demand from home-care workers are increasing, mainly as result of the expanding coordinating role they have to play.

There will be an estimated shortage of about 3,000 – 5,000 nurses in health-related social care and a shortage of several thousand workers qualified to level 3 of vocational training.

Poland: There has been a significant decline in the number of employees in the long-term care facilities operating in the health sector in the past few years, and this is forecast to rise in the next few years. This is due to the lack of new and young employees as well as the retirement of existing staff.

The forecast for the number of workers in the care-related professions by 2031, developed by the ENEPRI (European Network of Economic Policy Research Institutes) project team, is particularly negative for Poland. It indicates that while 650,000 people were employed in care-related professions in 2011, there will be only about 350,000 employees in these professions in 2031, close to half the current number.

Portugal: In general, there are no significant shortages of qualified and non-qualified workers in the labour market, due to the high numbers of unemployed. This employment situation will persist in the short to medium term. After that, it may improve at a modest pace, and so the current surplus in the labour market may persist for a considerable period of time.

Between 2008 and 2011, about 120,000 new jobs were created in Portugal, of which about 64,000 were in health and social care. At the same time, however, 480,000 jobs were lost. These figures suggest that future employment growth in the health and social care sector is estimated to grow by a few thousand jobs per year at most.

Spain：The Trade Union Confederation (Comisiones Obreras, CCOO) formulated two different scenarios for determining the number of new posts to be created under the framework of the System for Personal Autonomy and Dependency Care (Sistema para la Autonomía y Atención a la Dependencia, SAAD) in 2011 – 2015. In an ideal scenario, where all beneficiaries receive professional services, 261,007 new posts could be created, including staff in residences with accommodation, day centres and home-care.

In a more restrictive scenario—where 25% of dependent people would receive a financial subsidy for relatives to care for them, and the remaining 75% were assisted by professional services—a total of 195,755 new professional posts would be created, made up of 91, 202 posts in residences with accommodation, 45,360 in day centres and 59,193 in home-care services.

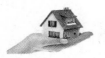

UK: As a result of population ageing and the increasing number of people with chronic illnesses and disabilities, the demand for social care services in the UK is projected to grow rapidly. It has been estimated that the number of jobs in adult social care in England will grow by between 24% and 82% between 2010 and 2025.

3. Labour market situation for care and support services

External factors influence the development of the labour market for care and support services for adults with disabilities or health problems. These factors may pose challenges to or offer solutions for labour market management. They can be identified by looking at the six domains specified in the PESTLE analysis: political, economic, social, technological, legal and environmental (see Annex. 1).

(1) Political and legal factors

The specific national political and legal framework of care and support services for adults with disabilities or health problems vary widely. Differences exist in relation to: (1) general care policy aims; (2) degree of centralisation or decentralisation; (3) the types of providers of formal care; (4) direct-payment systems versus provision of formal care services; (5) the funding structure.

Ⅰ. General care policy aims

Although the visions of home care formulated by central governments differ widely across Europe, according to the Home Care across Europe report, some common features can be found[①].

First, national governments' visions of home care are usually formulated rather generally and often do not define key concepts or specify measurable targets. Second, governments often foresee a growth in home care, usually designed to replace residential and hospital care. Third, the vision of home care generally refers to ageing societies and to users and their families' preference for home care. Home care is "adapted to the societal transformation"[②] and is seen to fit the goal of increasing the quality of life. In this context, many governments promote the independence of people with disabilities. Fourth, support for informal care-givers seems to be interwoven with the vision of formal home care, because home care is seen as a way of facilitating informal care. The vision of home care in many eastern European countries such as Bulgaria is furthermore entangled with employment policy. Some countries use this as a

---

① Genet, N., Boerma, W., Kroneman, M., Hutchinson, A., and Saltman, R. B. (eds.) (2012), Home Care across Europe: Current Structure and Future Challenges, Observatory Studies No. 27, World Health Organization, Copenhagen.

② Ibid..

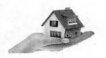

means of reducing unemployment, especially among women, by creating part-time jobs in home care. Fifth, better coordination between different types of home-care services is also mentioned as a goal in several policy documents, for instance in the UK. Sixth, other issues addressed by the policy documents include the level of quality of care and increasing the home-care workforce (such as in the UK and the Netherlands); increasing the role of civil society within home care (for instance, in the Netherlands and Portugal); and home care as a means to prevent or ensure early detection of social isolation.

In addition to this general picture, some country-specific developments in policies are detailed in the country reports. The main developments in general policies in the field of care and support services for adults with disabilities or health problems are summarised below.

Austria: A key objective of Austrian long-term care arrangements is to help individuals remain at home and live independently for as long as possible. This means that community-based care services will be further expanded in the future. Another priority is to formalise contractual arrangements between the care recipient and the care-giver, including (often undeclared) migrant carers.

Bulgaria: The transition to decentralisation of social service delivery in Bulgaria started in 2003 with legislative reform, supported by consistent policy measures. It is widely recognised in Bulgaria that the ageing of the population and the decreasing ability of family members to care for their elderly and disabled relatives will lead to a growing demand for community-based care services. These services are seen in the context of contributing to the independence of people with disabilities as well as improving the quality of life of their families.

Denmark: Home-care services in Denmark were introduced as a less-intrusive model of care. The provision of care was reframed as care for "health consumers" rather than care for "patients". The implementation of these new models took place in a decentralised governance structure, in which county and local boards became more important. This decentralisation in public administration accelerated the trend of deinstitutionalisation in Danish policies.

France: Partly as result of an ageing population creating more demand for care, the costs of the French care system are rapidly rising. Cost reduction policies are increasing the-already high-level of home and community-based care. Another rationale for encouraging community care is to stimulate the ability of patients to be independent for as long as possible.

Germany: Care policy is aimed at increasing immigration from countries outside the EU. A series of law amendments has been

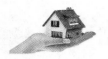

passed to facilitate the immigration of highly skilled workers and specialists to Germany. This will affect the community care sector. Qualified nursing personnel from outside the EU now have easier access to the German labour market.

The Netherlands: The Dutch cabinet considers community-based health and social care to be a top priority. Integral local made-to-measure care leads to better services for the citizen and to the early identification of problems. To this end, the new cabinet has continued the policy of increasing the level of community-based care ("extramuralising") and moving responsibility to community level. At the same time, the emphasis is on decreasing the demand for professional care by, for instance, focusing on sickness and disability prevention, self-management and informal care. More so than in the past, clients and their relatives are responsible for arranging care.

Poland: Currently there is no systematic approach to long-term care in Poland. However, adjustments to legislation are being prepared to improve this situation. These include plans to introduce vouchers with which families can purchase products and services needed for the care of family members, and an obligatory contribution to care insurance in the health protection sector.

Portugal: In Portugal, national policies are strongly influenced by ongoing public budget- and debt- consolidation processes and other measures to reduce the state's role as economic operator. Health, education and social care services are being rationalised, and the state's role as market regulator is being enhanced. In the next three to five years, these measures will reduce the availability of public resources to fund the welfare function of the state. This will put more pressure on private care-providers to support people in need and maintain appropriate quality standards and territorial coverage.

Spain: Given the current economic and financial crisis, the Spanish government has introduced several measures that indirectly affect the maintenance or creation of quality jobs in the care labour market. One of the most important changes is the labour reform approved in February 2012. The government strongly believes that its measures will help to maintain employment levels and that the most significant effects will be seen once the economy begins to recover. Furthermore, the Spanish Employment Strategy 2012 – 2014 highlights the importance of promoting employment in emerging economic activities such as the growing social and health sector, and particularly in activities linked to dependency.

UK: Several pieces of legislation are relevant to or have been instrumental in developing community-based care in the UK. The equal rights of disabled people in various areas of public life, with implications for social care providers in all sectors and the workforce, are being promoted. The independence, protection and

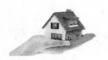

quality of care in the community is to be improved. Direct payments and personal care budgets are being introduced, enabling service users to exercise greater choice and control over their individual care needs. The government seeks to cut spending on residential care and reinvest these funds in community-based services, thereby increasing the use of direct payments and personal budgets.

II. Degree of centralisation

The degree of centralisation of policymaking and executive tasks in the field of formal care (the state versus regional or local authorities) varies. The Home Care across Europe report shows that policymaking responsibilities in home care are moderately decentralised in many countries. Policymaking on home healthcare tends to be more centralised than social home care. Governmental control is most centralised in Belgium, Cyprus, France and Switzerland and most decentralised in Iceland and Italy[①]. In a number of countries studied for this project-such as Austria, Bulgaria, Denmark and the Netherlands-the country correspondents report an increasing decentralisation of policymaking and executive tasks in the field of formal care towards lower-level authorities.

The conditions under which people are eligible for community-

---

① Genet, N., Boerma, W., Kroneman, M., Hutchinson, A., and Saltman, R. B. (eds.) (2012), Home Care across Europe: Current Structure and Future Challenges, Observatory Studies No. 27, World Health Organization, Copenhagen.

based care versus institutional care and the process of care assessment differ both from country to country and between the type of care, as the analysis of the country studies shows. In most of the countries studied, there are formal eligibility criteria for publicly financed community-based care services (except in Bulgaria for some types of community-based care).

Care assessment is mostly the responsibility of more localised authorities and organisations. In the Netherlands, however, the national Care Assessment Centre (Centrum Indicatiestelling Zorg, CIZ) decides on the exact eligibility criteria for personal care and home nursing within the boundaries of governmental guidelines.

(2) Providers of formal care

The providers of formal care vary from country to country and cover a wide range of organisations, including public institutions, private companies, third-sector organisations and NGOs such as churches and religious organisations. Usually, there is a mix of types of care providers. The situation in Portugal illustrates the great variety in types of providers.

(3) Community-based care in Portugal

Holy Houses of Mercy (Santas Casas de Misericórdia) :

These organisations have existed for centuries. Traditionally the

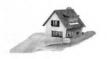

misericórdias provided basic health assistance to deprived people, but over time they have diversified their activities to supporting children, the aged and disabled people, delivering professional training and fighting social exclusion and unemployment. Though inspired by the Catholic Church, Portuguese misericórdias are not subject to its hierarchy.

Parochial centres and other religious organisations, such as the religious orders: Parochial centres are established by the bishop of the diocese of the church parish where they operate. The range of services provided by the parochial centres, which vary according to the size, degree of urbanisation and other local community factors, may include homes for the elderly, leisure-time and day-care centres, home and respite care services, pre-school and kindergarten centres, musical schools and other cultural, educational, sport, leisure, social and healthcare activities.

Mutualities or mutual benefit associations: Having their origins in the medieval brotherhoods, their first modern form was created in 1840 as a mutual credit institution. Mutualities are organisations that provide services to their members, notably in the supplementary social security area, such as health insurance, sickness and retirement pensions, subsidised health services and pharmacies, day-care centres and pre-school and kindergarten centres. They also provide concessionary loans, litigation assistance, scholarships, holiday centres and other services.

Cooperatives: These were started in the 19th century and developed significantly in the year following the military coup of 1974. Some cooperatives provide social and healthcare services.

Other not-for-profit institutions: These include foundations for social solidarity and volunteer associations for social action that actively provide social and healthcare services.

Commercial organisations: This grouping includes insurance companies, fund-management companies, operators of nursing and care homes and residential homes for the elderly and disabled.

Other providers: Alongside formal care organisations, individuals and families can be registered as providers of social care services. They are subject to similar regulations to those that apply to organisations and can benefit from the same incentives as the organisational providers. Three services fall into this category: child-care workers, family helpers and foster families for the elderly and disabled people.

Some countries have considerably less variety of care providers. For instance, in Denmark, the Netherlands and the UK, community-based care is mainly delivered by public institutions and private companies. In some of the countries studied for this report, such as Bulgaria, Poland, Portugal and the Netherlands, correspondents report an increasing outsourcing of care services to private providers.

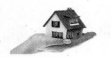

Ⅰ. Direct-payment systems

In all countries studied, care and support services are supplied by the state. There are also countries with direct-payment systems alongside the formal provision of services. Direct-payment systems give clients a personal budget with which they can purchase professional care themselves or pay family members to take care of them. Clients become, in a sense, employers.

Throughout Europe, the concept and implementation of direct payment appear to differ in a number of ways[1]: (1) entitlement rules, numbers and types of beneficiaries; (2) target groups, either client or the informal care-giver; (3) amounts of money (compared to benefits in kind) and the social rights linked to them; (4) procedures for testing eligibility and specific use of the budget, and for assessing the quality of services provided; (5) whether only cash benefits are available or there is a choice between benefits in kind or in cash.

Reported examples of countries with direct-payment systems alongside the provision of care services are Austria, Bulgaria, Spain, the UK and the Netherlands.

---

① Genet, N., Boerma, W., Kroneman, M., Hutchinson, A., and Saltman, R. B. (eds.) (2012), Home Care across Europe: Current Structure and Future Challenges, Observatory Studies No. 27, World Health Organization, Copenhagen.

II. Funding structure

The most common sources for the funding of these care and support services in European countries are: (1) taxation (may be collected at national, regional or municipal level); (2) insurance (can take different forms and be either compulsory or voluntary); (3) donations and other third-party contributions (care may be provided by charities or NGOs funded by private donations or membership fees, while some countries receive funding from the EU); (4) out-of-pocket payments (clients are required to pay a co-payment for care funded through taxation or social insurance).

Typically, funding consists of a mixture of these sources. Only in Denmark is taxation the sole source of funding[1].

In most of the countries studied in depth, tax-based public provision in the form of laws or national insurance provides allowances for long-term healthcare and social care. In some cases, people have to pay a part of the care costs themselves.

The funding structure in the 10 countries can be summarised as follows.

Austria: Austria has a mix of universal and income-related allowances and benefits in-kind.

[1] Genet, N., Boerma, W., Kroneman, M., Hutchinson, A., and Saltman, R. B. (eds.) (2012), Home Care across Europe: Current Structure and Future Challenges, Observatory Studies No. 27, World Health Organization, Copenhagen.

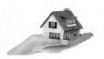

Bulgaria: Funding of social services in Bulgaria is based on a system of redistribution of public finances and is carried out in centralised and decentralised ways. The main sources of financing of social services are the state budget and the Operational Programme for Human Resources Development (OPHRD) (an ESF programme).

Denmark: The funding of the healthcare system is tax-based, which means that most services are free of charge and the main actors, both purchasers and most suppliers, are public. Legislation allows local authorities some limited freedom in setting charges for home help and some other non-health-related expenses.

France: Sources of funding are taxation and co-payments by clients.

Germany: Germany has implemented a public insurance system for nursing care that is based on the principle that the current contributions of insurance scheme members are used directly to finance the expenses of care-seekers (Umlageverfahren). Unlike a capital stock system, where individual contributions are saved and accumulated, the pay-as-you-go funding system has to finance new spending with an equal amount of revenues. Deficits thereby must be settled either by raising the government's debt or by changing the level of contributions.

Netherlands: The funding of the Dutch care system is partly tax-based, under the Exceptional Medical Expenses Act (Algemene Wet Bijzondere Ziektekosten, AWBZ) and the Social Support Act (Wet maatschappelijke ondersteuning, WMO) , and partly insurance-based. The Basic Health Insurance Act (Zorgverzekeringswet) covers the costs for family doctor, hospital and pharmacy. For other costs, people can pay into a supplementary health insurance. Community-based care for adults with disabilities is mainly financed by the AWBZ and WMO. In general, people also have to pay a part of the care costs themselves. Apart from public care, there is also private care in the Netherlands.

Poland: In Poland there are two main sources of funding for community-based care: public funds, partly insurance-based and partly tax-based, and private fees to businesses delivering long-term care.

Portugal: Besides proceeds from sales of goods and services, property income, private transfers (which include donations and legacies) and various other sources of income, a significant proportion of the revenue of the sector comes from government transfers and other public contributions and subsidies.

Spain: Generally speaking, public authorities are responsible for determining citizens' rights and deciding what services will be provided, and for assigning financial resources. The actual provision of services may be shared between public and private agents. The

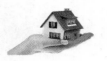

funding of the social services system in Spain as a whole is managed at three administrative levels, national, regional and local. The service user also pays part of the total costs, depending on their particular circumstances.

UK: Most funding for community-based care in the UK comes from central government through the Revenue Support Grant. The government also allocates specific grants to local authorities. A large proportion of spending comes from funds that local authorities raise themselves, primarily from the residence-based tax it levies. Local authorities are also expected to achieve significant savings in their budgets for social services in addition to undertaking commercial activities to generate income.

With the rise in demand for care and rising care costs, clients generally have to pay a larger share themselves. This can be seen, for instance, in the Netherlands and Germany.

The funding structures of specific labour market management initiatives also vary between countries. There are large budget differences between countries. Some countries, such as Bulgaria, are more dependent on EU funding from sources such as the ESF, while the northern Member States rely more on national funding.

(4) Economic factors

The care sector is an important economic sector and major

source of jobs. At present, all countries in this study are suffering from the effects of the economic crisis, some more than others. The crisis is affecting the community-based care labour market in different ways. In most countries, the health and social care sector is faced with cost-cutting measures. To some extent, these cost reductions limit the demand for labour in this sector. In the Netherlands, for instance, as a result of substantial cutbacks in social care there is less demand for social care workers. In the UK, social workers and carers employed by the local authorities face pay cuts and pay freezes. The private providers of care services commissioned by local authorities are also affected.

In less-prosperous times, the financial argument for community-based care above institutional care is even more important. This may lead to more demand for labour in community-based care, and less in institutional care.

On the supply side, the economic crisis makes the public care sector more attractive to work in than the private sector where the consequences of the crisis are generally much more far-reaching. This means more labour supply for community-based care. In Bulgaria, for instance, social care services are said to have become more attractive to those out of work as a result of the worsening labour market, characterised by an overall unemployment rate of 12%, and an unemployment rate among young people of 27% and of 45%

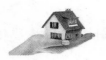

among the over-50s.

Cutting unemployment, and particularly youth unemployment, is usually high on the agenda during a financial crisis and labour market measures are more widely used. In this climate, it is possible that this may also make more labour available for community-based care. The Dutch cabinet, for instance, recently allocated 50 million extra for the years 2013 and 2014 specifically to combat youth unemployment. Half of the money is destined for the "School Ex" programme to encourage intermediate vocational-level students to continue with their studies, especially in areas with labour shortages such as healthcare. The other half of the government money is allocated to local schemes organised by municipalities and the Dutch employment service to help young people to find a job. In addition, a Youth Employment Ambassador (Aanpak Jeugdwerkloosheid) will be appointed.

(5) Social factors

I. Sociodemographic factors

First, the most important sociodemographic factor influencing the community-based care labour market is the rapidly ageing population. The number of older people (65 years and older) in the EU27 plus Norway and Switzerland is expected to increase from 89 million in 2010 to 125 million in 2030[①].

Second, Figure 3 compares the expected development of the old-age-dependency ratio in the EU27 with that predicted in the 10 countries studied. This indicator is the ratio between the total number of elderly people at an age when they are generally economically inactive (65 and over) and the number of people of working age (15 to 64 years of age).

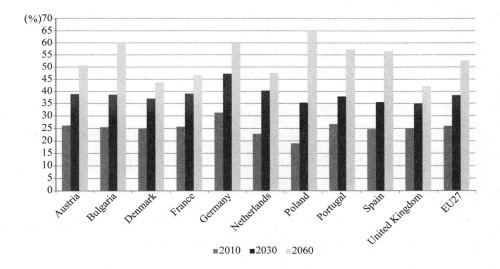

Figure 3   **Old-age dependency ratio predictions for the EU27 and**

the 10 countries

Source: Eurostat.

---

① Rodrigues, R., Huber, M. and Lamura, G. (eds.) (2012), Facts and Figures on Healthy Ageing and Long-term Care, European Centre for Social Welfare Policy and Research, Vienna.

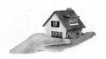

In the EU27 as a whole, the old-age dependency ratio is expected to increase from 25.9% in 2010 to 38.3% in 2030 and 52.6% in 2060. This increasing trend is also true for the 10 countries studied here, though the growth pace differs.

In 2010, the ratio is highest in Germany, Portugal and Austria (respectively 31.2%, 26.7% and 26.1%) and lowest in Poland, the Netherlands and Spain (19.0%, 22.8% and 24.7%). In 2060, the ratio is predicted to be highest in Poland, Bulgaria and Germany (respectively 64.1%, 60.3% and 59.9%) and lowest in the UK, Denmark and France (42.7%, 43.5% and 46.7%).

As more people live longer and the number of people with dementia, chronic illnesses and disabilities rises, the demand for care workers increases. At the same time, the ageing of the population leads to a dwindling supply of labour.

Other sociodemographic factors influencing the community-based care labour market are the decline in the number of young people as a result of lower birth rates and the appearance of new family models.

As a consequence of lower birth rates, the entry of young people into vocational training will fall. The Dutch national report notes that in the Netherlands there seems to be a trend of young people entering preparatory higher education instead of preparatory vocational training. This suggests that in the future the availability of workers with higher-level qualifications in health and social care in the Netherlands will grow, but there will be shortages of nurses at the vocational level.

Lower birth rates will also reduce the availability of people in the younger generation (working in other economic sectors) to take care of their own elderly relatives. This will reduce the availability of informal care, increasing the demand for formal care and people to staff it.

Another sociodemographic factor, explicitly reported for Spain, is the emergence of new family models, such as growing numbers of single-person households and more widespread participation of women in the labour market. This means that fewer women will be available to provide informal care and the need for formal care will increase.

II. Sociocultural factors

Sociocultural factors influence the labour market for care and support services for adults with disabilities or health problems. An important factor in this respect is the proportion of formal care versus informal care. As the Home Care across Europe report shows, in the majority of EU countries informal care-givers such as family, neighbours and friends provide an estimated 60% of the home care individuals need on average[1]. In Greece and some central European

---

① Genet, N., Boerma, W., Kroneman, M., Hutchinson, A., and Saltman, R. B. (eds.) (2012), Home Care across Europe: Current Structure and Future Challenges, Observatory Studies No. 27, World Health Organization, Copenhagen.

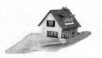

countries, for example, 90% of home-based care is provided by families. In contrast, only 15% of the home-based care is given by family members in Denmark.

Figure 4 provides detailed information on the degree of formalisation of care in relation to the labour intensity of the care sector. The left part of the figure shows the percentage of the care sector workforce in relation to the total population aged 65 and above. The right part shows the ratio of the care sector workforce in relation to the users of formal care services aged 65 and above. The latter indicator can also be seen as a proxy input indicator of the quality of care. Higher scores mean higher levels of formalisation in relation to labour intensity.

The following conclusions may be drawn from Figure 4: (1) the left side of the figure shows that the degree of formalisation of care arrangements is reflected in the relative importance of the long-term care workforce in relation to the old-age population. Norway, Denmark and Sweden are examples of de-familialisation, where the satisfaction of welfare needs are becoming independent of the family and instead a responsibility of the State, although the latter has recently shifted back to greater family responsibility. (2) The right-hand side of Figure 4 shows how the ratio of the workforce in relation to the older population benefiting from care services is related, to

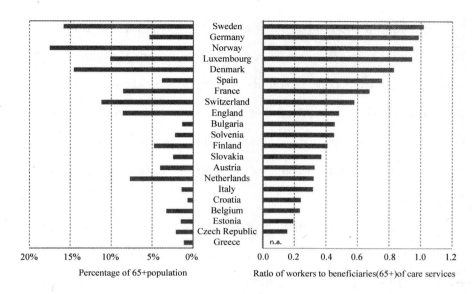

Figure 4　People formally employed in the care sector as a % of those aged

　　　　65 and older（left）and ratio of people formally employed in the

　　　　care sector to service users（right）

Notes: Data for France refer to 2003 and 2008.

Source: Rodrigues, R. , Huber, M. and Lamura, G. (eds.) (2012) , Facts and Figures on Healthy Ageing and Long-term Care, European Centre for Social Welfare Policy and Research, Vienna.

some extent, to care services or expenditure as detailed in the previous chapter. There are, however, differences caused by the prevalence of part-time work (for instance, in the Netherlands) and the importance of cash benefits that can be used to pay for family members or migrant care workers (as in Austria or Italy)[1].

---

① Rodrigues, R. , Huber, M. and Lamura, G. (eds.) (2012) , Facts and Figures on Healthy Ageing and Long-term Care, European Centre for Social Welfare Policy and Research, Vienna.

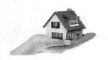

In some of the study countries, such as Austria and Bulgaria, a recent shift towards formal care can be seen. In Austria, for instance, informal care by family members is declining. This is due to societal change as the number of working women is rising and is estimated to increase further. Professional nursing and care services are becoming more important to support the balancing of work and family life.

More or less the same development can be seen in Bulgaria, where deep attachment to home and family is traditional. However, social change has made it difficult to devote oneself to the family, especially in cases where family members are seriously ill and dependent. If a person has to care for an ailing relative, they must leave their job, which lowers the quality of life for the whole family. Institutional long-term care, despite being very much against Bulgarian tradition, then becomes a feasible solution. Therefore it is socially justified and effective for the state to financially support the home-based care of people who have families and homes, paying their relatives to care for them.

However, in other countries, such as the Netherlands, policies have moved towards more informal care, with the emphasis on decreasing the demand for professional care by, for instance, promoting prevention of sickness and disabling conditions, self-management and informal care. The relatives of clients are increasingly responsible for arranging their care.

A drawback of informal care is that people delivering care to disabled relatives are wholly or partially removed from the labour market.

III. Socioeconomic factors

A third relevant category is socioeconomic factors. As already mentioned, the economic crisis has had a significant impact on the health and well-being of citizens. The particularly poor economic situation in some countries may lead to an increase in health and social problems, thereby increasing demand for care workers.

(6) Technological factors

Technology has brought important developments to the health and social care sector.

Higher life expectancy, as a result of advances in medical knowledge and treatments, will lead to a greater demand for long-term care in the future. Also, the likelihood of getting severe illnesses usually increases with advancing age. As a consequence, not only the demand for care personnel in general but also the demand for more highly qualified care personnel is expected to rise.

Labour productivity in community-based care has increased, although gains are comparatively low. In theory, the increasing deployment of assisted-living technology, such as domotics (home

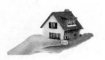

automation), telecare and digital participation services, and innovations in materials used in personal care, such as dry washcloths, have led to more efficiency, higher labour productivity and thus less labour demand in community-based care. The recent CARICT (a contraction of "care" and "ICT") research project, conducted by the Institute for Prospective Technological Studies (IPTS), shows that there is a wide range of successful, not very costly, and beneficial examples of ICT-based support for carers across Europe[1]. However, the sector is and will remain comparatively labour-intensive. Also, experience in the Netherlands, for instance, shows that technological innovations have a greater influence on the quality of care than on the labour productivity of care workers.

The increasing use of assisted-living technology by clients will have implications for the home-care workforce. Development of new skills will be required to assist people with the use of such technologies. For instance, in the UK, Skills for Care is working towards providing the home-care workforce with comprehensive and practical guidance on the skills, knowledge and understanding related to assisted-living technologies that social care staff in a

---

① Carretero, S. , Stewart, J. , Centeno, C. , Barbabella, F. , Schmidt, A. , Lamontagne-Godwin, F. and Lamura, G. (2013), Can technology-Based Services Support Long-term Care Challenges in Home Care? Analysis of Evidence from Social Innovation Good Practices across the EU, CARICT project summary report, Joint Research Centre of the European Commission, Publications Office of the European Union, Luxembourg.

variety of community-based roles will need to have. The deployment of assisted-living technology in the UK also has led to the introduction of a new type of home-care worker, the assistive technology support worker.

(7) Environmental factors

A final PESTLE domain is the environment. The influence of this factor on the care labour market, however, may be considered negligible. This goes for most of the 10 countries studied. Only in Portugal does the environmental sector increasingly provide opportunities to develop social and meaningful jobs to assist the integration of unemployed adults with disabilities.

4. Labour supply

While the demand for care-givers is on the rise, the supply of workers is decreasing due to an ageing workforce. In Denmark, France, the Netherlands, Spain and the United Kingdom, about a third of care workers are over 45 years old[1]. The European

---

[1] Korczyk, S. (2004), Long-term Workers in Five Countries: Issues and Options, AARP Public Policy Institute, Washington DC. Ewijk, van H., Hens, H., and Lammersen, G. (2002), Mapping of Care Services and the Care Workforce: Consolidated Report, Working Paper No. 3, Thomas Coram Research Unit, Institute of Education, University of London.

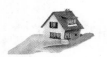

Commission estimates that between 2000 and 2009 the number of health and social care workers over the age of 50 increased by 20%[1]. Personnel replacement needs will lead to 7 million job openings up to 2020 (in addition to 1.4 million new jobs)[2]. The Commission expects that this mismatch between labour supply and demand will lead to a shortage of 2 million healthcare workers in 2020, of which 1 million will be long-term care-givers. Hence, in 2020 Europe is expected to be 8.5% short of the required number of healthcare workers.

5. Employee characteristics

The surveys and reports referred to above also highlight several characteristics of the health workforce. Firstly, the health and social care workforce in the EU27 consists primarily of women. Secondly, compared to the total workforce, the health and social care workforce is relatively highly educated, at least in the EU15. When the new

---

[1] European Commission (2012), Towards a Job-rich Recovery, COM (2012) 173 final, Brussels.

[2] Korczyk, S. (2004), Long-term Workers in Five Countries: Issues and Options, AARP Public Policy Institute, Washington DC. Ewijk, van H., Hens, H., and Lammersen, G. (2002), Mapping of Care Services and the Care Workforce: Consolidated Report, Working Paper No. 3, Thomas Coram Research Unit, Institute of Education, University of London. European Commission (2012), Commission Staff Working Document on an Action Plan for the EU Health Workforce, SWD (2012) 93 final, Strasbourg.

Member States are included, the percentage of workers with higher vocational or university education in the sector decreases to the average in the overall economy.

The high educational level of the sector's workers is also reflected in the workforce forecasts. From the 8 million healthcare jobs that are expected to be created in 2010 – 2020, most will be given to highly educated personnel (5 million), then to personnel with medium-level qualifications (3 million), and only 0.2 million jobs are expected to go to personnel with low-level qualifications.

The ratio of part-time workers in the health and social care sector is also much higher than in the overall economy, 31.6% compared with 18.8% respectively. A notable feature is the relatively low pay for health and social care workers. The Commission notes that even though the skill levels are relatively high and working conditions are often demanding, hourly wages in the sector as a whole are lower than the average hourly wage of the total EU27 workforce. In recent years, this tendency-which is related to the high rate of female employment in the sector and to the gender pay gap-has become more pronounced[1].

---

[1] European Commission (2010), Second Biennial Report on Social Services of General Interest, SEC(2010) 1284 final, Brussels.

Chapter Three : Recruitment and Retention Measures

This chapter discusses the results of the analysis of the 30 recruitment and retention measures studied in depth for this project. It explains the classification of these measures according the labour market strategy they support, and then briefly describes policies and actions in this area at national level. An overview of the main elements of the 30 recruitment and retention measures selected is presented[①].

---

① The criteria for selection of the 30 cases were described in the introduction. The annexes to the country reports contain full descriptions of the case studies.

1. Type of recruitment and retention measures

By distinguishing between measures that stimulate the supply of labour and measures intended to temper the demand for labour, it is possible to categorise possible solutions to labour shortages in the sector. Using the solutions model (described in Annex 1) as a starting point, four labour market strategies addressing recruitment and retention in community-based care to support adults with disabilities can be identified.

First, targeting labour reserves to attract new employees to the sector. In addition to the recruitment of the unemployed and other groups currently not working in community-based care, this may also include targeting existing immigrant groups and labour migrants.

Second, promoting and facilitating the education of potential employees through, for instance, the creation of new and specific learning paths, the launch of campaigns to encourage people to choose an educational path in the sector and institutional improvement of the connection between the labour market and education in general.

Third, improving the situation of current employees to optimise their potential as well as to discourage them from leaving the sector. This may include the introduction of training and retraining

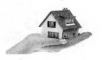

programmes, professionalising the sector and providing more career prospects for existing employees.

Fourth, improving the operational management and labour productivity of organisations in the sector. This could be a way of alleviating labour market discrepancies by allowing organisations to work more efficiently and increase the productivity of their employees, for example through the use of new technologies and treatment methods, and changes in functions and organisation. The labour intensity of community-based care work makes it difficult to increase efficiency, but innovative approaches may nonetheless have a positive impact.

2. Policies and actions at national level

The analysis of the country reports shows that in most countries there are initiatives in each of the strategies described above. However, the emphasis varies. Some countries, like Poland, focus more on improving the overall quality of social care, thereby improving the quality and attractiveness of care jobs. Denmark and Finland also focus on raising the prestige of the sector. In countries where the general quality is already fairly high, like the Netherlands, the focus is more on targeting new labour reserves and improving productivity. The UK is drawing more people into the lower levels of the sector. There are also large differences in the specificity of the initiatives. In Portugal, for example, most labour market initiatives are targeted broadly, although care jobs are often a priority, while Spanish initiatives are more narrowly focused on jobs in home care.

The analysis of the country reports also reveals interesting similarities between countries. Many have developed telecare projects (the Netherlands, Spain and the UK), increased the number of migrant care workers (Austria and Denmark), changed the organisational structure of care (Bulgaria, the Netherlands and Spain) and introduced new direct-payment systems (Austria, Bulgaria, the Netherlands, Spain and the UK).

3. Case studies : Good practice in recruitment and retention

This section presents an overview of the main elements of the 30 recruitment and retention measures studied in depth. For the purposes of the study, the cases are classified according to the most important strategy they address (sometimes cases address more than one strategy).

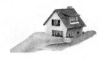

(1) Strategy 1 : Targeting labour reserves

This strategy primarily aims to recruit home-care personnel from labour reserves, especially the unemployed. Initiatives are a combination of professional orientation, prequalification, qualification, work experience, mediation and follow-up support and labour cost subsidies.

Labour Foundation for Social Work and Healthcare Professionals (Austria) : This initiative targets unemployed people in Vienna interested in a job in health, nursing or care work, or in the social work professions. It helps them to train for and then find a job. Candidates go through a multistage selection procedure in the workplace whereby they will ultimately be employed after finishing their training, being selected on the basis of criteria such as personal suitability, motivation and language proficiency. The coordinating organisation is the Vienna Employment Promotion Fund, and it pre-selects applicants.

Migrants Care (Austria) : The Migrants Care initiative prepares people with a mother tongue other than German for jobs as qualified health and social-care workers. Within the framework of the initiative, interested migrants are informed about the possibilities of jobs in community-based care and are counselled individually. They can take part in prequalification training with a focus on German language skills to make it possible for them to progress to vocational training in the field of health and social care.

Assistants for disabled people (**Bulgaria**) : The dual goal of this national programme is to provide work for the unemployed and to provide community-based care for those who need it. The programme finances two types of care jobs. The personal assistant role is designed to ease the situation of families who have a disabled relative in need of constant care, while the social assistant role is intended to meet the daily needs of people with disabilities or of severely ill and isolated people, including the organisation of their leisure time to improve their social inclusion. Relatives of disabled people can apply for the role of personal assistant.

Job Rotation (**Denmark**) : The Job Rotation initiative is intended to improve the professional development of current employees and, at the same time, provide access to employment in community-based care for the unemployed or newly qualified workers. The jobs of current employees undergoing training are held open for them and temporarily filled by unemployed people. This initiative therefore combines work experience for the unemployed (Strategy 1) with upgrading the qualifications of current personnel (Strategy 3, described below).

Stimulus 2012 (**Portugal**) : Stimulus 2012 grants financial support for the recruitment and training of job-seekers who have been

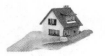

registered as unemployed for more than six months. It subsidises 50% of the salary of those employed under the scheme for a maximum of six months. An additional subsidy of 10% can be granted for certain categories of job-seeker, including those who themselves have some kind of disability. Employers who have claimed the subsidy have to offer a permanent employment contract or a renewable fixed-term employment contract for at least six months after the scheme ends.

Employment/Inclusion (Plus) (Portugal): The Employment/Inclusion (Plus) programme offers job-seekers temporary employment in the social services for 12 months; it targets job-seekers in disadvantaged groups such as the long-term unemployed particularly. The primary aim is to improve the future employability of job-seekers by maintaining or enhancing their personal and professional skills, by keeping them in touch with the labour market and by reducing their sense of isolation and demotivation.

Single Ticket Programme (UK): The Single Ticket Programme (STP) operating in Manchester targets unemployed people and people from disadvantaged groups, offering an opportunity to gain knowledge, skills and experience of working in health and social care. The main criteria for the selection of participants are commitment and willingness to work in health and social care rather than previous experience or academic qualification in this sector. The approach of the STP's vocational training is to help workers gain core skills and experience of a wide variety of career choices through one comprehensive programme—a "single ticket". The aim is to create flexibility in the workforce. The programme consists of 4 weeks of induction training and 5 work placements, each of about 12 weeks' duration, with health and social care providers. These could be in adult care, child care, mental health, in a general hospital or working with people with learning disabilities. Participants who complete the programme should have a solid basis to apply for a permanent job in the sector.

(2) Strategy 2: Promoting and facilitating education

This strategy is intended to recruit health and social care students and retain them in the sector. The aim is to provide a larger supply of qualified school-leavers who are able and willing to work in the community-based care sector. The examples of this strategy can be divided into three subgroups: campaigns and educational orientation, apprenticeships in health and social care, and mentorships.

I. Campaigns and educational orientation

Boys' Day (Austria): During the annual Boys' Day, boys can get acquainted with professions in care and education presented

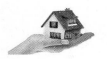

by male role models. The long-term objectives of the Boys' Day are: (1) to bring more men into typically female professions; (2) to break social stereotypes; (3) to improve the image of the social work and healthcare professions; (4) to support boys in developing a positive male identity.

In addition, throughout the year, job-orientation workshops are held for schoolboys aged 12 and over, where they are shown films about work in the social sector and on social culture. The initiative also has its own website.

Care4future (Germany): The Care4future initiative ran between 2010 and 2011 and aimed to address the shortage of skilled labour in the care sector by informing, sensitising and inspiring adolescents at secondary school stage to consider a career in the care sector. It resulted in the development of a manual on how to set up local or regional networks of people involved in the care sector and a framework for a training course to be delivered by members of the network. It also introduced a peer-learning approach to training, in which trainees from nursing schools become lecturers for secondary school students. This approach is combined with a two-week internship in a care facility in which students are mentored by current senior staff.

Ⅱ. **Apprenticeships**

Neighbourhood Training Company (the Netherlands): The

Neighbourhood Training Company is a new concept in practical community-based training for health and social care. It helps trainees to acquire work experience that is directly connected to their training in healthcare and welfare work in their own residential district. They carry out odd jobs that residents cannot do for themselves and for which they do not receive help from their municipality.

INOV-SOCIAL (**Portugal**) : The INOV-SOCIAL initiative gave financial assistance to professional apprenticeships in social care for new graduates from higher vocational education, usually for nine months. The main objectives of this initiative were to complement or enhance the professional skills of the graduates and to facilitate their integration into the social care labour market, and also to improve the quality of the services provided.

Ⅲ. Mentorships

Mentoring for students with a foreign background (**Denmark**) : This system offers mentoring to health and social care students from non-Danish ethnic backgrounds to encourage them to complete their education, to reduce drop-out rates and to offer better preparation for careers in community-based care. In the mentoring system, each student is paired with a mentor. Mentors are health and social-care teachers or volunteers who are either still working in the sector or have recently retired. The mentoring system is coordinated by a network that arranges work experience and acts as a contact

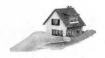

point between mentor and student.

(3) Strategy 3: Improving the circumstances of current employees

The third strategy is intended to prevent current employees from leaving the sector, either by improving their qualifications or by offering them other routes towards professional development. Although this is the primary aim, upgrading the community-based care sector also makes it more attractive to potential employees and contributes to the recruitment of personnel. Measures adopted under this strategy may include: professionalising the sector; offering training and retraining programmes to increase knowledge, skills, competences and motivation and at the same time providing more career prospects for employees; and taking alternative or more modern approaches to training and education, such as e-learning and professional validation of work experience.

Ⅰ. Professionalising the sector

Professionalising staff development in the care sector (Germany): This initiative ran from 2009 to 2012 and aimed to develop managerial skills in parts of the care sector workforce, for instance in the field of human resource development. Extra occupational courses were offered to equip participants with knowledge that was as practice-oriented as possible. Courses combined theoretical management seminars with the implementation of an on-the-job project. The initiative also aimed to raise awareness within the community-based care services of the need for systematic and strategic human resource development. Human resource consultants were placed in nursing schools to advise the community-based care services on human-resources-related problems and to assist in the design of systematic human resource development.

New professional role for social workers (Poland) : This project developed a new social work standard, referred to as the "community organising model", which describes how social workers can support individuals, social groups and local communities threatened with poverty, marginalisation or social exclusion and can help to reintegrate them into the community and into employment by working with them more directly. Coupled with the standard is a financial incentive for social workers who have direct client contacts and who work in accordance with the standard. In 2013 – 2014, about 3,000 social workers will be given training in the new standard in a two-day course delivered nationally.

Social Care Workforce Development Programme (SCWDP) (UK) : This programme is a regional initiative offering grants to local authorities in Wales to develop a SCWDP partnership for their area. These partnerships are responsible for the development, planning, monitoring and evaluation of SCWDP-

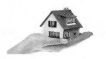

funded training across the public and private social care workforce in the area. They also develop the recruitment and retention strategies of social care providers by offering training on recruitment and retention matters to their management staff. The ultimate aim is to increase the proportion of staff with the qualifications, skills and knowledge they need and, in this way, to improve the quality and management of the social services provision in the area.

II. Training employees

Social Assistant and Home Assistant Service (Bulgaria): In Bulgaria, funds were available between 2007 and 2012 to increase the skills and motivation of social assistants and home assistants who were supporting dependent people with disabilities or people who were simply living alone and needed help. This three-phase programme primarily aimed to upgrade the skills of workers in the sector, both unemployed and employed, who already had experience in social work. The overall objective was to enhance and improve the social assistant service and to develop the home assistant service as a form of community-based social service for people excluded from regular social contact and at risk of becoming dependant on institutional care. The specific objectives of the programme were the creation of new jobs in the social services sector for professionals looking for additional work and increasing the skills and motivation of all social assistants and home assistants.

Further education in chronic disease (**Denmark**): To manage the high and increasing incidence of chronic diseases in many European countries, the skills of professionals in community-based care need to be upgraded. This Danish initiative is intended to enhance career development for health professionals in general practice, community-based care and hospitals. It includes a number of courses and training modules to increase the ability of the existing workforce to manage chronic disease in community-based care, with stronger links to clinical practice. The premise of the programme is that skills development should be offered on an intersectoral basis, through a team-based chronic disease management approach that is person-centred and tailored to individual needs.

Qualifications as the key to the improvement of care service quality (**Poland**): This project in the Wiekopolska region of Poland concentrated on the training of people already active in long-term care, the majority of them in some formal role. Training, in the form of lectures as well as practical experience, covered methods of care for the elderly, disabled and those with health problems, among other topics.

Ⅲ. New approaches to employee education

Professional accreditation for experience of working in community-based care (**France**): The French system of professional accreditation on the basis of experience (Validation des

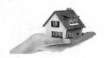

Acquis de l'Expérience, VAE) enables individuals with at least three years' work experience to get a professional qualification or diploma. VAE is open to those who can prove they have a salaried job, are self-employed or are voluntary workers. Candidates have to document their relevant work experience, answer questions on the qualification to be awarded and take an oral exam. The certification procedure is organised by various ministries, each responsible for establishing that candidates fully meet the requirements for VAE in their sector.

E-learning in the care sector (eLiP) (Germany): The eLiP (eLearning in der Pflege) initiative aims to boost the diffusion of e-learning in the care sector, by providing a central e-learning infrastructure that individuals can access at a reasonable price. Rather than opting for the e-learning offerings that were already available on the market, the eLiP project managers believed that a software solution tailored to the care sector would gain acceptance and widespread use in the sector.

Professionalism certificates (Spain): In the Spanish system of professional validation by experience, each professionalism certificate is made up of a number of "competence units", normally two or three, each of them directly linked to a short training module. A partial certification for each unit is needed to get the overall professionalism certificate. The contents, competence units, professional contexts and profiles of the professionalism certificates are officially regulated by royal decrees approved and published at national level. The Ministry of Labour and the Ministry of Education are the main national bodies responsible for the process. Autonomous communities and their labour and education authorities are responsible for the implementation of the accreditation system at regional level.

(4) Strategy 4: Improving management and labour productivity

Innovative changes in functions, organisation or applied technology, or any combination of these three factors can improve the operational management and labour productivity of the community-based care sector. Besides cutting labour costs, new ways of working can make the sector more attractive to current and potential employees, and so increase the possibility of recruiting and retaining personnel. Cases that illustrate the use of this strategy can be divided into four subgroups according to the kind of changes made: new functions; new ways of organising and steering care activities; technological innovations; and new employment and transport services for adults with disabilities to help them participate more actively in the labour market, education and society in general.

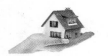

Ⅰ. New functions

Visible Link（the Netherlands）：Between 2009 and 2012, this programme promoted the cost-effective deployment of highly skilled district nurses, especially in neighbourhoods with socioeconomic and health disadvantages. The role of the district nurse is to address citizens' problems, and particularly those in vulnerable groups, by connecting them with various authorities and organisations at district level in the fields of housing, prevention and health and social care. As well as coordinating healthcare and social care, nurses also provided care themselves in people's homes. The primary aim of Visible Link was to improve the coherence of care at district level.

New profession of medical carer（Poland）：This measure introduced vocational training for the new profession of medical carer in long-term care. Under the supervision of nurses, medical carers carry out simple nursing tasks originally performed by qualified nurses. This new profession has been included in the list of professions（the Polish Classification of Occupations and Specialisations）kept by the Ministry of National Education, and after completing the relevant vocational training, medical carers can now be officially registered.

Ⅱ. New ways of organising and steering care activities

Netherlands Neighbourhood Care（the Netherlands）：This

project gives small, self-organising district teams of highly skilled workers full responsibility for the nursing and care of clients at home. These teams can enhance the services available to clients by supporting the contribution of volunteers or by helping clients to access the formal health and social care system. When necessary, they provide home nursing or care themselves. These local teams are supported by a small and efficient national organisation. The objective of the approach is to improve the quality and efficiency of home care and make the job of district nurse or orderly more attractive.

Independent Life (**Spain**): Independent Life is a direct-payment project in the Gipuzkoa region aimed at promoting autonomous and independent living for disabled people over 18 living in their own homes. Beneficiaries autonomously manage their own care budgets and are responsible for recruiting their personal assistants, whether relatives or qualified professionals. Each beneficiary employs on average two to three personal assistants to give them support with daily tasks they cannot do on their own. The disabled person supervises this support and the personal assistant does not take over decision-making.

SSI Group (**Spain**): The SSI (Servicios Sociales Integrados, Integrated Social Services) Group is a non-profit cooperative of social care professionals in Bilbao. The cooperative model of the SSI

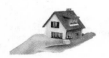

Group is characterised by self-government, self-management, equal participation, collective property, communication and cooperation, and a decentralised human resource structure. Other essential values are personal growth, continuing training, the maintenance of professional standards, the support of social initiatives and the reinvestment of the benefits they accrue in society. One of the aims of the SSI Group is to support informal carers to achieve formal qualifications and, in doing so, to increase the value of their work.

Ⅲ. Technological innovations

Assistive Technology Norfolk (UK): This project is aimed at developing a new type of social worker specialised in assistive technology: the assistive technology (AT) support worker. AT support workers carry out assessments of (potential) services users, such as stock-taking of wishes and needs as regards assistive technology, whether standalone or telecare equipment. They also take care of subcontracting the installation of the equipment and provide training, awareness-raising sessions, talks and clinics around the county for various groups.

Ⅳ. New employment and transport services for adults with disabilities

Social Entrepreneurship (Bulgaria): Between 2009 and 2011 the Social Entrepreneurship grant scheme aimed to create new models of successful social enterprises and to improve existing ones.

By doing so, the objective was to create secure jobs, especially in the service sectors, for vulnerable groups not able to participate in regular work. The programme facilitated and supported social enterprises, raised awareness and stimulated cooperation between parties involved in this field.

Establishment and service supports through work (ESATs) (France): The state-funded ESATs (Etablissements et Services d'Aide par le Travail) aim to find work for people whose disabilities are too severe for them to work in normal organisations or even disability-friendly organisations. By integrating workers with disabilities into society, the medical and social workers of the ESATs become part of a network of local partners and are able to source housing, preventive medicine programmes, care and even cultural activities for their clients. They therefore both provide work for people with disabilities and support them in life outside work to promote their social inclusion.

PMR transport service (France): The PMR (Personnes à Mobilité Réduite) transport service in Grenoble uses minibuses that are able to carry up to five people in wheelchairs and are fitted with floor rails to secure them. The PMR driver-carers make door-to-door journeys but do not help people in and out of their home. If necessary, other carers help before and after the PMR service. The PMR driver-carers, mostly men, are specially trained: they take a

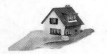

first aid training course, and courses in smooth and preventative driving and in the handling of wheelchairs. They have regular training with disability professionals to appreciate better the various disabilities they encounter and learn how to deal with passengers during the journey.

Chapter Four: Outcomes, Results and Impact

In general, the information on outcomes, results and impacts of measures aimed at recruiting and retaining care workers is fragmented. Eastern European countries especially do not have a long-standing tradition of consistent and regular evaluation. Programmes and projects in other European countries are not always evaluated either. It is, however, usually obligatory for beneficiaries of EU funds such as the ESF to carry out evaluations.

In addition, many of the initiatives in place are still in operation and can therefore be only partially evaluated. It should also be noted that, in general, assessing the net effects of labour market policies on staff shortages is not always easy. This has been confirmed by a recent Dutch feasibility study on the difficulties of

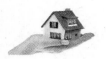

evaluating labour market measures in the healthcare sector[①]. The book shows that, in the short term, the impact of only some labour market initiatives on current or expected staff shortages can be adequately assessed. In the long run, a larger part can be more fully evaluated. However, since the influence of external factors will always increase over time, the reliability of such assessments will be limited. The quality of available data would also have to be improved to make a more accurate impact assessment possible. Even so, some quantitative aspects (such as effects on productivity and the reach of labour market measures) and qualitative aspects (such as bottlenecks and the identification of success or failure factors) can usually be evaluated.

1. Case studies: Outcomes

Most of the 30 cases studied have been monitored or evaluated, either in quantitative or more qualitative terms. In general, the outcomes and results of the initiatives are promising. However, it is difficult to compare the outcomes, results and impact of the various initiatives with each other, as they differ in matters such as aim,

---

① Panteia, SEOR and Etil (2013), Effectmeting van arbeidsmarktmaatregelen in de zorgsector. Een haalbaarheidsstudie [Effects of labour market measures in the healthcare sector: A feasibility study], Panteia, Zoetermeer, the Netherlands.

strategy, scope, regional scale and duration. Furthermore, different indicators are used for measuring success. Job creation is not the direct aim of all the initiatives, nor is information always available about the number of jobs created. In some cases other indicators are used, such as the number of people reached by a measure, the number of places available, the number of people actively participating and the number of people successfully completing it.

This part of the report presents an overview of the outcomes of the 30 case studies. The results and impact of the initiatives are then briefly discussed.

(1) Outcomes of Strategy 1: Targeting labour reserves

Labour Foundation for Social Work and Healthcare Professionals (**Austria**): Between January 2003 and September 2007, 740 home helps, 206 nursing assistants and 20 certified health carers and nurses completed vocational training; 95% of this group found a job. After 9 to 12 months, the employment rate of this group remained at about 90%.

Migrants Care (**Austria**): Approximately 350 people called in to the central contact point, which was open from July until September 2012. Many were helped with a short, informative conversation. Around 200 comprehensive and individual counselling sessions took place. Due to budget constraints, only one

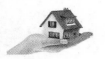

prequalification course for 18 people was held in 2012.

Assistants for Disabled People (**Bulgaria**): More than 80, 000 jobs were created by the programme between 2005 and 2011.

Job Rotation (**Denmark**): In 2012, some projects were still under way, with an estimated 770 participants placed in temporary positions. Out of a group of 291 job-rotation temporary workers who completed a rotation project, 78% were employed within two weeks of the end of the project. In addition, 63% of a group of 286 temporary workers were employed two weeks or more after the rotation was completed, compared to 43% of a comparison group that had not been enrolled. The increased satisfaction and growth opportunities for existing employees in the sector suggest that retention has been successful, although there are no data to confirm this.

Stimulus 2012 (**Portugal**): The measure has already attracted a significant number of beneficiaries: of the 3,231 organisations and 5,547 jobs approved by October 2012, 487 (15%) organisations and 1, 006 (18%) jobs pertained to the social care sector. In addition, there were 528 new jobs for activities related to care services for the elderly and people with disabilities, more than half of which (52%) were for social workers.

Employment/Inclusion (**Plus**) (**Portugal**): In 2011, 55, 1038 unemployed people were covered by this measure, of whom 3,

478 were delivering social care services to elderly people. In 2012 (up to September), 44,788 unemployed people were covered, with 3,581 providing social care to the elderly. There is currently a trend of increasing participation by social care services in tender procedures, possibly explained by the downturn of economic activity the country is experiencing.

Single Ticket Programme (**UK**): Since 2009, around 70 people participated in the programme. On completion of the programme, around 70% of participants have gone on to secure work positions in health and social care.

(2) Outcomes of Strategy 2: Promoting and facilitating education

Ⅰ. Campaigns and educational orientation

Boys' Day (**Austria**): During 2011, more than 4,000 boys throughout Austria took part in Boys' Day: 1,522 boys from 50 schools attended a total of 111 workshops; 2,375 boys from 112 schools visited 153 facilities in the education and care sectors; and 102 boys from 26 schools participated in individual sample placements in 96 facilities.

Care4future (**Germany**): No quantitative information was available.

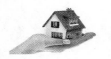

II. Apprenticeships

Neighbourhood Training Company (the Netherlands):
Neighbourhood Training Company activities started in the cities of Dordrecht, Haarlem, Hengelo, Leiden and Utrecht in 2011, and each have between 15 and 22 trainee positions. The project in the Hague, which started in January 2010, has nearly 100 trainee positions. Other cities and regions running Neighbourhood Training Company projects include Amersfoort, Rotterdam, Veenendaal and Zuid-Kennemerland.

INOV-SOCIAL (Portugal): In 2010, 1,050 trainees took part and in 2011, 1,467. Up to September 2012, when the measure was replaced, there were still 219 trainees who had benefited from it.

III. Mentorships

Mentoring for students with a foreign background (Denmark): Beginning with 15 pairs in 2004, the programme had up to 100 pairs by 2010, and at present there are 50 mentor-student pairs. Of the students surveyed, 70% stated that their mentor has been a significant support for them in finishing their educational programme; 46% of the managers of funded projects reported that the mentorship system has resulted in more young people with immigrant backgrounds successfully completing their academic programme.

(3) Outcomes of Strategy 3: Improving the circumstances of current employees

Ⅰ. Professionalising the sector

Professionalising staff development in the care sector (**Germany**): So far, 180 participants from 150 community-based care services have participated in one of the courses.

New professional role for social workers (**Poland**): In the initial phase, 82 social workers took part in the project. It is expected that 3,000 social workers will participate in the dissemination training in the period 2013 – 2014.

Social Care Workforce Development Programme (**SCWDP**) (**UK**): In 2010 – 2011, up to 127,000 people attended SCWDP-funded events, a decrease of 3.8% on the previous year. Some 6,500 qualifications were gained during the year, a decrease of 2.9% on the previous year. The number of "specified qualifications" obtained in the training areas of management and community-based care decreased slightly (6% and 4% respectively). There was a 14% increase in child-care qualifications.

Ⅱ. Training employees

Social Assistant and Home Assistant Service (**Bulgaria**): In total, 4,152 social assistants and 6,785 home assistants were

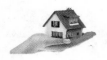

employed within the framework of the three phases of the grant scheme.

Further education in chronic disease (Denmark) : The goal of the project was to train 3,000 people between 2010 and 2012; however, 5,834 people participated.

Qualifications as the key to the improvement of care service quality (Poland) : The project attracted 330 participants.

Ⅲ. **New approaches to employee education**

Professional accreditation for experience working in community-based care (France) : Among the 51,000 candidates who applied for VAE in 2011, almost one in three were applying for certification of vocational training recognised as a qualification for carers and home-care auxiliaries. Of these, 6,300 applied for a state-recognised nursing auxiliary diploma; 4,800 applied for a state-recognised home-care social assistant diploma; and 1,900 applied for a qualification as a home-care family assistant.

eLiP (Germany) : eLiP started with seven members in 2008. In 2012, the association had 20 members who all make use of the e-learning infrastructure and participate in introductory and advanced seminars offered by eLiP.

Professionalism certificates (Spain) : A total of 787 people completed the requirements for the professionalism certificate in health and social care services for dependent people in households in the summer of 2012. Just over 57% of those who entered the initial assessment phase were awarded the certificate. Within social services and community services, 1, 634 gained the professionalism certificate in health and social care for dependent people in social institutions, and 1, 202 gained the certificate for care delivered within a household setting. Within the health professions, 352 people gained the professionalism certificate in health transport.

(4) Outcomes of Strategy 4: Improving operational management and labour productivity

Ⅰ. New functions

Visible Link (the Netherlands): The target was to recruit 250 extra district nurses. During the mid-term review in the spring of 2011, a total of 95 district projects were running in 50 municipalities. At that time, the projects had recruited approximately 355 extra employees. Of these, 250 were district nurses with higher vocational training levels (71%), 75 were district nurses with intermediate vocational training levels (20%) and about 30 were employees from other disciplines such as social workers (9%). Jobs for project managers were also created. Given that during the mid-term review not all the projects had completed the recruitment and selection phase, the final number of extra district nurses and other employees within the Visible Link initiative will certainly be higher.

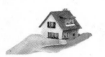

New profession of medical carer (**Poland**) : No quantitative information was available.

Ⅱ. New ways of organising and steering care activities

Netherlands Neighbourhood Care (**the Netherlands**) : This initiative started with one self-steering district team in the city of Almelo in 2006. By 2012 the number of teams had reached 470 , up from 360 in 2011. The number of employees in district teams was 5 , 500 in 2012 , up from 3 , 700 in 2011. The average number of employees recruited yearly has been around 1 ,200.

Independent Life (**Spain**) : When this regional programme started in 2004 , only four individuals were involved. Eight years later , 39 people were taking part in the programme. It is estimated that each beneficiary generates on average 2 or 3 personal assistant positions , suggesting that the number of jobs created is between 78 and 117.

SSI Group (**Spain**) : According to the 2011 annual report , SSI Group had a total of 320 workers. The majority of them (99%) were women. At the end of 2012 , the total number of staff in the group had increased to 400 – 450 people.

Ⅲ. Technological innovations

Assistive Technology Norfolk (**UK**) : The AT service worker team has grown from 6 to 13 members in the past few years. From the original six AT service workers , one person left (due to ill-health).

There have not been any staff reductions as a result of introducing the assistive technology service.

IV. New employment and transport services for adults with disabilities

Social Entrepreneurship (**Bulgaria**): As a result of the programme, 29 new social enterprises were set up and 10 existing ones were supported. The total number of people covered by the project in 2012 was 3,612 from various risk groups, of which 1,606 are disabled. More than 140 people were engaged in the delivery of social and medical services. These were predominantly part time and temporary jobs.

ESATs (**France**): In 2001, ESATs had 25,500 employees. In 2006, there were 1,345 ESATs, with 29,000 employees providing medical, social and employment support for some 110,000 disabled people.

PMR transport service (**France**): A survey conducted in 2007 in 65 major urban areas showed that these services employed 700 people, 80% of whom were drivers. In Paris, more than 1.6. million journeys a year are made using these services.

2. Results and impact

On the basis of the analysis of the country reports, the following

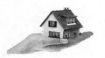

overall conclusions about the results and impact of the initiatives can be made. (1) In most cases the quantitative targets of the initiatives were reached or are expected to be reached. The approaches chosen usually function well in practice or at least prove to be relevant. (2) The initiatives have positive labour market effects, contributing to job creation, recruitment and retention of personnel. They also combat unemployment and staff shortages. (3) There are also social gains: the initiatives contribute to the social inclusion of unemployed people and the empowerment and quality of life of vulnerable citizens, and assist social cohesion within communities.

In addition, as the country reports show, most initiatives studied are either expected to be or have already proven to be sustainable and transferable to other organisations or regions in the same country. In some cases, they have already been taken up in other countries and organisations.

These positive results are partly due to the context (the PESTLE factors, as described in Chapter Two), which offers a favourable environment for community-based care, and certainly also to the intrinsic characteristics and qualities of the initiatives (see the discussion on success and failure factors in Chapter Five).

Chapter Five: Lessons Learnt: Success and Failure Factors

This chapter focuses in detail on what can be learned from the 30 recruitment and retention initiatives discussed in the previous two chapters. It identifies the success and failure factors associated with the initiatives; these are classified and examined according to the four strategies of the solutions model. Lessons on the sustainability of the initiatives and of their transferability to other regions, countries and sectors are also discussed.

1. Lessons from Strategy 1: Targeting labour reserves

(1) Employment programmes for unemployed job-seekers

Most European countries have employment programmes for

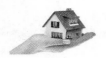

unemployed job-seekers in the health and social care sector. These programmes offer benefits to the different stakeholders: (1) unemployed people gain the necessary qualifications for paid work; (2) employers get qualified employees to fill their vacancies; (3) clients receive the care they need; (4) the costs of unemployment are reduced.

Usually, the programmes comprise vocational training or work experience or both. In some cases there are also labour cost subsidies for employers.

(2) Recruitment, selection and prequalification

Before unemployed job-seekers can be trained, they have to be recruited, selected and—in some cases—prequalified by various means.

First, preferably they are recruited not only through large-scale labour market information campaigns, but also through personal consultations with job-seekers. Second, prioritising traditionally disconnected segments of the labour market, such as the long-term unemployed or people with an ethnic background, contributes to achieving broad integration objectives. Third, reaching specific target groups of labour reserves such as the migrant population demands a specific target group approach. In the Migrants Care initiative (Austria), the personal counselling-in which the eligibility and motivation of the migrants are assessed and a realistic insight in the future field of work is given-turned out to be an important success factor. Fourth, the importance of a good, careful selection procedure in employment programmes for unemployed job-seekers is highlighted by the Labour Foundation for Social Work and Healthcare Professionals (Austria) and the Single Ticket Programme (UK). Not only the candidates but also their future employers have to be selected carefully. Fifth, financial incentives for unemployed job-seekers can remove barriers to participation in employment programmes. For instance, the beneficiaries of the Employment/ Inclusion (Plus) programme in Portugal are given supplementary payments and keep their other subsidies or benefits.

(3) Vocational training

The following success and failure factors are apparent in the vocational training of unemployed job-seekers.

First, good vocational education institutions are just as important as good candidates. In the Austrian Labour Foundation initiative, the results of the different education institutions are monitored. Comparing the quality of educational institutions has been shown to improve the standard of vocational training. Second, using officially regulated, acknowledged curricula contributes to acceptance by employers. Third, the set-up of the vocational training of unemployed

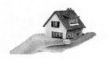

job-seekers is important. The UK Single Ticket Programme, for instance, consists of four elements: a unique recruitment process; an intensive four-week induction; five separate work placement modules of approximately 12 weeks each in the area of health and social care, providing five different references and thus giving a stronger basis for a permanent job application; and a nationally recognised qualification for those who complete the programme. The fact that the programme is offered free of charge can also be seen as a success factor. Possible failure factors in this case include the need for participants to travel to various work placement locations, finding enough organisations offering work placements, finding suitable people within these partner organisations who understand the programme's ethos and the resistance of some current employees within these organisations to change. Fourth, in a number of cases, the participants of vocational training programmes are guaranteed a job beforehand. Sometimes, their future employee is also known. This stimulates the candidate to finish the training course successfully and also means that training can be fine-tuned to the wishes and needs of the employer.

(4) Work experience

Gaining work experience can also contribute to enhancing the labour market opportunities of unemployed job-seekers. Success factors for the Job Rotation initiative (Denmark) turned out to be job interviews with the unemployed beforehand, guidance by a supervisor in the workplace and the prospect of being supported in further education after the end of a period of temporary employment under the scheme.

(5) Mediation and follow-up support

Where vocational training or work experience is done without the guarantee of a job on completion, or when trained candidates are not taken on by employers who had previously promised work, there is a need for mediation. For instance, the Austrian Labour Foundation scheme has been supplemented by a placement service.

In some cases, employment projects targeted at unemployed people lead to fixed-term or part-time jobs, and these situations would seem to demand some kind of follow-up support for the new employees. In practice, however, follow-up support is generally not available.

(6) Labour cost subsidies

In general, financial incentives for employers, such as labour cost subsidies, turn out to be an effective labour market measure. Usually, the primary aim of labour cost subsidies is to create jobs for less-privileged job-seekers. Stimulus 2012 in Portugal does not oblige

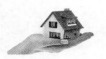

an employer to offer a permanent employment contract, and this may be seen as the main success factor of this measure. The level of subsidy makes it worthwhile for employers, as does the fact that they are allowed to combine it with other measures available. This also contributes to the success of this initiative.

(7) Formalising non-formal employment

The case studies also offer examples of formalising previously non-formal employment. For instance, relatives of disabled people can apply for inclusion in the Assistants for Disabled People scheme in Bulgaria. The Independent Life direct-payment scheme (Spain) enables people with disabilities to gives contracts to personal assistants, who may or may not be relatives, as they choose. One of the explicit aims of the cooperative SSI Group (Spain) is to qualify informal carers and, in doing so, to increase the value of their work.

2. Lessons from Strategy 2: Promoting and facilitating education

(1) Campaigns and educational orientation

First, in many European countries, generalised campaigns aim to raise awareness among young people about the care sector and the courses and careers available. However, specific groups require a targeted approach. The success factors evident in the Boys' Day initiative (Austria) include tailoring the nationwide initiative to the local context and the continuation of activities all year round, such as marketing, films and job-orientation workshops for schools, designed to maintain the awareness created by the initial Boys' Day events. The workshops are seen as a particularly effective element of the Boys' Day initiative.

Second, the Care4future initiative in Germany shows that professional orientation in the community-based care sector can be improved by building up and maintaining a local or regional network, and by offering a blueprint for training courses that can be offered by members of the network.

Third, the successful transfer of knowledge in this initiative relies on a peer-learning approach, in which trainees become teachers for secondary school students, combined with a two-week internship in a care facility during which students are tutored by senior mentors. The atmosphere is more informal and open to discussion, and the information is presented in a humorous manner which eases and increases knowledge transfer.

(2) Content and set-up of education

First, the content and set-up of health and social care education have to be carefully considered. Courses must be attractive to the

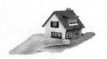

students involved, but at the same time appropriate for the needs of their future employers.

Second, emphasis on practice rather than theory is preferable, along with learning on the job. For underprivileged students such as migrants and those with low-level qualifications, intensive coaching and individual attention are important.

Third, important success factors in the mentoring of health and social care students with ethnic backgrounds (Denmark) are the network of mentor coordinators, their contacts and collaboration with the schools and the support of the schools. Another success factor is the correct matching of student and mentor. The two parties have to have similar expectations, the age difference cannot be too big, and it helps if they are based near each other. A failure factor can be mentors who lack sufficient time to counsel their students because they have work commitments.

(3) Trainee posts

Trainee posts bridge the gap between education and the labour market. Attractive trainee posts contribute to the motivation of the students involved and encourage them to finish their studies successfully, to move on to a higher level of education and perhaps to choose a career in the community-based care sector. Furthermore, they contribute to a better match between the training provided by educational institutions and the needs of employers.

An important success factor in community-based, practical training, as adopted by the Neighbourhood Training Company initiative in the Netherlands, is the made-to-measure approach in which a special "labour broker" is deployed to match the right student with the right client.

A success factor in the INOV-SOCIAL measure (Portugal) was the "merchandising" of work in the social care sector to students by raising their awareness of the sector and to social care institutions by interesting them in offering apprenticeships. A failure factor for this initiative was the relatively high administrative burden and cost. There is also a thin line between an apprenticeship provided to help a young graduate to enter the labour market and a wage subsidy to reduce an employer's labour costs. This might create an incentive to abuse such initiatives by engaging trainees without much consideration of their need for personal development.

3. Lessons from Strategy 3: Improving the circumstances of current employees

The situation of current employees in community-based care may be improved by professionalising the sector and upgrading employees' qualifications and skills. Means of doing this include

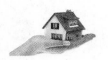

regular training programmes, professional validation by experience and e-learning.

(1) Professionalising the sector

Professionalising community-based care is, first and foremost, about developing and enhancing standards for work and workers in the sector. An example of this is the development of the role of social workers in Poland using the community organising model.

Establishing and maintaining partnerships with the objective of developing the sector's workforce facilitates professionalisation at regional and local level. The partnerships in the framework of the SCWDP (UK) are a good example of this. A failure factor here, however, was the slightly controversial role of the SCWDP as a supporter of private providers. But attitudes towards privately-funded care services have changed over the years. The majority of care services are now contracted out to independent sector providers, and very few services are directly provided by local authorities.

Equipping professional care-givers with the skills for additional management tasks also contributes to the professionalisation of the sector. The initiative to professionalise staff development in Germany incorporated a practical component into the course that turned out to be a crucial success factor. It gave human resource consultants in the nursing schools an entry point into the management of the care service. This had the positive effect of raising awareness of the need for more professional management of community-based care.

(2) Training employees

Developing skills by training or retraining employees improves the quality of community-based care services. At the same time, it contributes to personal and professional growth and job satisfaction. Employees become more confident in managing new responsibilities, which enhances their employability, opens up more career possibilities and enables them to move higher up the pay scale. Retraining community-based care employees in an attractive setting not only contributes to their personal and professional development, but also to their motivation to continue to work in the sector.

An important success factor in the Danish initiative to develop the skills of healthcare staff in chronic disease management is the deployment of guest teachers from practical work environments, making the courses highly practice-oriented. Other success factors in this case are small class sizes (allowing participants to engage in dialogue with other sectors), regular evaluation and continuous adaptation of the courses to participants' needs and wishes. A failure factor-related to the intersectoral approach chosen for in this initiative—is the challenge of differentiating the courses to meet the specific needs of participants from different sectors.

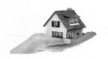

The Social Assistant and Home Assistant Service grant scheme in Bulgaria was intended to increase the skills and motivation of social assistants and home assistants through introductory training, supportive training and supervision. This design turned out to be a success factor.

The Polish initiative to improve the qualifications of care workers also points to the importance of an attractive and adequate training set-up. Success factors include classes in venues with modern equipment and training by enthusiastic, skilled care workers who are able to motivate the participants. Barriers to participation in training can be the cost and the travelling distance to the training facilities.

As a rule, employees prefer to train during working hours. For employers, this can be a barrier because employees undergoing training during working hours are not productive. The Job Rotation system (Denmark) solves this problem by allowing unemployed people to temporarily take over the work of employees in training.

(3) Professional validation of experience

Professional validation of experience can be defined as a system in which knowledge, skills and competences gained through work experience or non-formal methods of training are acknowledged with professionalism certificates. Examples are the professionalism certificates initiative in Spain and the system of professional accreditation based on work experience in France. Both schemes promote the professionalisation of the community-based care sector and improve workers' qualifications and, in doing so, facilitate the mobility of the labour market in the sector, clarifying the nature of the skills held by its workers. In the French system, the relatively low cost of the accreditation of work experience compared to conventional vocational training, since workers are productive while training on the job, is seen as an important success factor. A failure factor is the written nature of the assessment procedure. A move towards more practical tests would undoubtedly benefit more candidates with weak writing skills. Systematic professional support would also improve the success rate of accreditation procedures.

(4) E-learning

E-learning interactive training using a network-connected computer-has cost advantages. The other main arguments for deploying e-learning in the community-based care sector include：(1) more options for vocational and continuous education of employees；(2) flexibility；(3) easy adaptation to individual learning pace；(4) reduced travel time and costs；(5) attractiveness to young people.

The CARICT research project described in Chapter Two

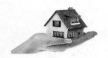

supports these arguments.

The eLiP initiative (Germany) shows that the presence of a sufficient number of workstations at an employer's facilities contributes to the success of e-learning. It also shows that the further away conventional education facilities are, the better the acceptance of e-learning. A failure factor is that older decision-makers and teachers may be sceptical about e-learning, being less familiar with electronic media than younger people.

4. Lessons from Strategy 4: Improving operational management and labour productivity

Besides reducing labour costs, measures to improve operational management and labour productivity through new ways of working can contribute to the attractiveness of the community-based care sector for current and potential employees, and so improve the conditions for recruiting and retaining personnel.

(1) Innovation in functions

Creating new types of functions can improve efficiency in community-based care. One possibility is "job carving", a way of splitting jobs to ensure that the most suitable person carries out each task. In this way new functions can be created. It is a flexible way of managing a workforce that allows employers to use the skills of staff in the most productive way, and also enables less able workers, such as those with disabilities, to make a valuable contribution to the world of work. In Poland, formalising the new profession of medical carer by registering it in the official list of professions contributed to the success of the initiative.

Another way to improve the efficiency and attractiveness of work in community-based care is to give professionals in the field greater responsibility and autonomy. The new-style district nurse introduced by the Visible Link initiative in the Netherlands, that added more coordination functions and scope for initiative to the traditional role of these health professionals, turned out to be highly attractive to the existing staff.

(2) Organisational innovations

Changing the organisation or management of care activities by, for instance, applying concepts such as self-directing district teams and cooperatives can enhance the operation of community-based care.

The preconditions for self-directing teams that function well, like those created by the Netherlands Neighbourhood Care initiative, include: (1) the ability of the team to make its own decisions within a clear framework, agreed upon with the management; (2) the well-

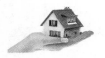

balanced composition of the team, good relations within it and mutual agreement on the division of tasks; (3) regular solution-oriented meetings to discuss work, in which decisions are reached by consensus; (4) joint responsibility for organisational tasks and outcomes, with clear agreements about who is available and when, to prevent overburdening team members with work, particularly in the set-up phase.

The cooperative model of the SSI Group (Spain) is characterised by self-management, participation and collective property, communication and cooperation, and a decentralised human resource structure. Other essential values are personal growth, training and professionalism, and social initiative. This collaborative model is the main success factor of the SSI.

Direct-payment programmes, in which the client effectively becomes the employer of their care workers, also change the traditional organisation of care delivery. The case study on the Independent Life programme in Spain illustrates the success and failure factors in this approach. Success factors regarding the management and functioning of this programme include: (1) fine-tuning of the support to the specific needs of the beneficiaries through an ' action protocol' that evaluates these needs adequately and assigns an appropriate amount of money for them to spend on care; (2) ensuring that agreement is made between the client and the personal assistant directly without interference from local authorities; (3) putting emergency measures in place to cope with exceptional situations, such as when none of an individual's personal assistants is available.

The successful recruitment and deployment of personal assistants seems to be more likely if relatives or close friends are not employed in the position, and by having several part-time assistants instead of one full-time assistant. The assistants need to be aware that the disabled person is capable of making their own decisions and, in turn, the "employer" needs to clearly define the tasks expected of the assistant from the very beginning. Ideally an "independent life plan" is set out, where all care and assistance needs are described in full, in order to define the personal assistants' work. Finally, it helps if the beneficiaries of the programme can organise themselves to support each other and share lessons learnt.

(3) Technological innovations

Technology can improve the operation of community-based care by providing innovative support systems at home, which help disabled and elderly people to live in their own homes. Technological solutions tend to be more cost-efficient and are effective in providing social and health support. They also reduce the need for the presence of relatively scarce health and social-care workers.

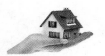

This has been confirmed by the CARICT project[①]. Deployment and use of technological services for informal carers is still limited, mainly due to users' limited digital skills, the lack of examples of such services in real-life settings, and the poor evidence for the impact and sustainability of these services. The CARICT project aimed to collect evidence-based results on the impact of ICT-enabled care services in the home, and to make policy recommendations to develop, scale and replicate them in the European Union. The methodology was based on a mapping of 52 ICT-based services for informal carers developed in Europe, and a cross analysis of 12 of these initiatives to gather data on their impacts, drivers, business models, success factors and challenges. The main results show that there is a wide range of successful, not very costly and beneficial examples of ICT-based support for carers across Europe. The cross analysis indicated that these services had positive impacts on the quality of life of elderly people and informal carers, the quality of care and the financial sustainability of the health and social systems.

Important success factors for the Assistive Technology Norfolk project (UK) included the support for the initiative within the organisation, regular awareness-raising and training, and the person-

① Cedefop (European Centre for the Development of Vocational Training) (2012), The Role of Qualifications in Governing Occupations and Professions, Cedefop, Thessaloniki.

centred approach of the AT support workers providing equipment tailored to individual needs. There were also some barriers, and these included: (1) the attitudes of social service professionals within the organisation, some of whom saw assistive technology as an add-on rather than a core service; (2) an assumption within the organisation that older people would not understand the new technology; (3) the perception of clinicians that the services posed a threat to their jobs; (4) the lack of a recognised formal qualification for the skilled staff installing and managing these systems.

(4) Employment services for adults with disabilities

Employment services for adults with disabilities not only aim to guide them into a paid job, preferably in the regular labour market, but also to give them continuing support when they do have a job. In some of the case studies examined by this report, adults with disabilities form a specific target group for employment programmes alongside other groups such as the long-term unemployed, the older unemployed and the migrant population.

Social enterprises offer an opportunity to improve the quality of life and social inclusion of vulnerable groups, including adults with disabilities, through active participation in the labour market. The case study of the Social Entrepreneurship grant scheme in Bulgaria identifies some failure factors which may occur when attempting to

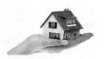

stimulate employment through social enterprises, such as the economic crisis, which reduced demand for the services of social enterprises, the lack of awareness of the social economy among the public and difficulty in accessing the target groups.

Policy is increasingly directed towards placing adults with disabilities in jobs in "disability-friendly" companies in the regular labour market, supported by job coaches if necessary. While sheltered work environments continue to be supported in many European countries, they are intended only for adults who cannot work in the regular labour market.

One of the problems faced by the ESAT facilities in France is that they compete with one another. The demands made by the government for improvement in their efficiency could have a negative effect, driving ESAT facilities to take on only disabled workers who have a higher level of productivity and to reduce the number of individuals who are less efficient in the work environment. Certain ESAT facilities are finding it hard to adjust to the demand for improved performance and more professional management. In the future, some may have trouble surviving financially once state subsidies are no longer enough to balance the accounts.

(5) Transport services for adults with disabilities

Special transport services enable less mobile adults with

disabilities to actively participate in society, for instance by transporting them to educational facilities or workplaces. Many public transport systems are working on better accessibility for people with disabilities, but there are still problems, especially on journeys from home to public transport systems in conurbations. Additional special transport services for people with limited mobility can help them get from their homes to their destinations on a regular or occasional basis. By having specialised vehicles and driver-carers, the transportation needs of disabled people can be met, aiding their social inclusion.

An example of a transport service for disabled adults that trains its drivers in social care is the PMR transport service in Grenoble, France. The service is a success, and its passenger numbers-and employment for driver-carers-are steadily increasing. Factors in this success include an increase in the number of people with limited mobility living independently and the decrease in authorisations for medical transport as a result of public cost-cutting.

5. Lessons learnt : Sustainability and transferability

The sustainability of successful recruitment and retention measures in care organisations is important, as is the transfer of lessons learnt from successful initiatives into other contexts.

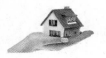 More and Better Jobs in Home-care Services

Examination of the 30 different case studies suggests a number of general observations that can be drawn about the sustainability and transferability of recruitment and retention measures.

(1) Sustainability
I . Political and public support

The political will to formulate policies and dedicate resources to the care sector is a crucial element of sustainability. Although this may seem self-evident, political willingness to act is rooted to a large degree in how important the electorate finds the proposed policies; when public opinion sees value in a particular policy direction, dedicating resources to that policy is legitimised.

In the case of care jobs, a number of case studies refer to the importance of political willingness and motivation of governments and municipalities to continue supporting a new measure. It is therefore important to make sure the public is aware of the growing needs of the care sector, as well as the increasing role it plays in society, if political interest is to grow and contribute to the sustainability of care-sector initiatives.

A number of measures try to do precisely this. Boy's Day in Austria aims to promote the view that working in healthcare is a worthy and rewarding profession and to get the message across that the care sector has a growing need for workers. The Care4Future

250

programme in Germany has a very similar goal.

In other countries, there is a need to change cultural attitudes about the care of disabled and elderly people. In Bulgaria, for instance, where caring for vulnerable relatives at home is seen as demanding for family members, limiting their freedom to work, the number of policies aimed at community-based care and the rate of transfer from institutionalised to community-based care are both rather low. This is gradually changing, however, as a different mentality towards caring for vulnerable groups is beginning to take hold. In Spain the situation is similar: attitudes towards caring for disabled or elderly relatives are altering gradually. Community-based care is coming to be viewed as an issue that society as a whole must work towards. The Spanish Independent Life programme demonstrates the importance of political willingness to sustain the measure. In Poland, new attitudes to social care have revitalised the care sector.

II. Funding

A second critical element in the sustainability of measures is the availability of adequate funding. In the majority of the cases in this study, funding comes from a combination of various public bodies such as municipalities, national governments and the ESF. In several cases this is combined with contributions from beneficiaries of the measures, be they companies, smaller social care and healthcare organisations, or clients. In any case, the majority of the initiatives

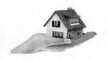

require finance and subsidies from the public sphere. Given the current economic climate in Europe, this brings their sustainability into question. This means that political willingness to continue funding such projects is essential.

A number of countries are encountering this particular problem. In Germany, Denmark and Bulgaria, the uncertainty of funding is a barrier to sustainability. In Germany, the eLip initiative is self-sustaining since the members of the information network pay a fee. Most measures require more financial input than this, however, and self-sustaining measures may be difficult to formulate.

Ⅲ. Cooperation and collaboration

Sustainability is affected by the presence or absence of two elements that go hand in hand: sound collaboration and coordination between the individuals and organisations involved.

In planning and implementing measures, the perspectives of all relevant participants are important so that expertise and insights from organisations are incorporated into any initiative. This will maximise the effect of the measure and the satisfaction of those involved. A fruitful measure that ultimately benefits both the service providers and the beneficiaries is more likely to be sustained. This point was apparent in various countries; the case studies from Denmark, France and Spain in particular demonstrated the importance of such collaboration.

A specific means of promoting collaboration and cooperation is the establishment of information and communication networks. A number of case studies demonstrated the value and usefulness of creating databases of client information to promote efficient and effective collaboration between the organisations involved.

The Netherlands Neighbourhood Care initiative relied on the use of an IT infrastructure to report on and plan the visits and duties of care workers. The German eLiP project was based around the notion of a shared IT network to promote learning amongst care workers. Spain's professionalism certificates also relied on a database that pooled information on clients for the various organisations and government bodies involved to make the awarding of qualifications as efficient as possible. Bulgaria also utilised a system promoting better communication with clients of the Assistants for Disabled People programme to greatly reduce potential inefficiencies and failure factors in providing care to disabled people.

Ⅳ. Transferability

It is important that a given country's existing social support and healthcare systems are taken into account when considering the transferability of a measure that originated there. In France, for instance, disabled people benefit from a number of allowances that are viewed there as important for improving social care; these measures alone may not provide sufficient support in other national

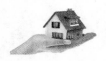

contexts. Observations from Poland also indicate that the success of any measure will depend on the legal and political frameworks in which it operates.

It would seem, however, that transferring a measure within its country of origin tends not to be too problematic. A number of case studies demonstrate that measures can be transferred to different regions and municipalities of a country, and to different care or labour contexts. Different regions of a country may have differing demands for social care and healthcare and will therefore have different levels of labour supply and demand. However, adapting to these factors is feasible.

A majority of the case studies suggest that the measures described can be transferred to different contexts. Bulgaria's Social Entrepreneurship grant scheme could be transferred to target groups with different disabilities or care needs. Denmark's Job Rotation scheme and mentoring for students with a foreign background could both be applied to different subsets of the labour market. Poland's initiative to improve the qualifications of care workers could also be applied to other professions. Austria's Boy's Day has already been applied to other professions. The Dutch Neighbourhood Training Company scheme could be used to generate experience for young people in other professions as well.

Some initiatives could potentially be transferred across national borders where the legal and political frameworks underlying them are simpler. Most of the case studies from Portugal, for instance, used simple subsidies, and so where there is political willingness in other countries, the INOV-SOC and Stimulus 2012 initiatives could be implemented with relative ease. Austria's Boys ' Day has already been implemented in Germany. The Netherlands Neighbourhood Care idea has also already been implemented in other countries because it does not rely on combinations of other social care and healthcare initiatives.

Chapter Six : Conclusions and Policy Pointers

1. Conclusions

At the centre of this study is the issue of job creation, recruitment and retention in community-based care for adults with disabilities or health problems. A functioning, sustainable and high-quality system of community-based health and social care provision is essential for European societies and economies. At the same time, this sector offers a lot of job opportunities. To overcome barriers to job creation in the sector, such as budgetary constraints and demanding working conditions, and to support the creation of a strong and growing workforce in the sector, many countries are already pursuing different recruitment and retention measures. This study examined 30 examples of good practice in 10 different countries from which other countries can learn.

In the 10 countries studied, the proportion of institutional care for adults with disabilities compared to non-institutional care varies widely. However, there is an increasing tendency towards provision of non-institutional care. The momentum towards home care appears to be driven by lower costs, policies promoting the greater independence of people with disabilities, the preferences of clients and the potential of assisted-living technology.

Generally, the labour market in the care and support sector offering services for adults with disabilities is characterised by staff shortages, especially at higher qualification levels. From the perspective of the care workers themselves, there are qualitative discrepancies because their terms of employment and working conditions are generally not good. The sector has an image problem, partly because of the objective problems surrounding poor terms of employment and working conditions, but also partly because of the subjective perception that caring is not a high-status occupation.

At the moment, the workforce shortages are temporarily mitigated by the economic crisis. In the longer term-with a continuing rise in the demand for long-term care as the population ages and a fall in the supply of labour as European economies recover-increasing shortages are to be expected. Innovative technological developments could lead to higher labour productivity in home-based care, but it is

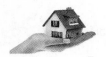

likely that this will remain a labour-intensive sector.

To combat the labour market discrepancies described above, four overall strategies can be identified: (1) targeting labour reserves; (2) promoting and facilitating education for potential employees; (3) improving the circumstances of current employees; (4) improving the operational management and labour productivity of organisations.

The 10 countries studied have initiatives in each of these categories, although the emphasis varies. In total 30 innovative approaches, all of which have been put into practice and have proved useful in recruiting and retaining home-care personnel, were documented and assessed for this report. In each of the four labour market strategy areas, different types of projects were selected. They include those that target: (1) labour reserves-professional orientation, qualification and prequalification, work experience, mediation or follow-up support, labour cost subsidies; (2) education-labour market communication campaigns and educational or professional orientation, apprenticeships in health and social care, mentorships; (3) current employees-professionalising the sector, training and retraining programmes, new approaches to training and education through, for instance, e-learning and professional validation by experience; (4) operational management and labour productivity-new functions, new ways of organising and directing care activities, technological innovations, new employment and transport services.

In general, the outcomes and results of the 30 case studies are promising. The initiatives have positive labour market effects such as contributing to job creation, recruitment or retention of personnel. There are also social gains since many assist the social inclusion of unemployed people, or empower vulnerable citizens and improve both their quality of life and social cohesion in their neighbourhood. Finally, most initiatives studied have already proven to be sustainable and transferable to other organisations or regions of the same country. In some cases, transfers to other countries may also be successful, and some have already taken place.

2. Policy pointers

Analysis of the 30 case studies identified a number of success and failure factors for the recruitment and retention of home-care personnel. On the basis of this analysis, a set of policy pointers related to the four labour market strategies are presented. These are followed by policy pointers on the sustainability and transferability of successful measures and a number of more general policy pointers.

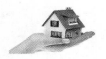

(1) Strategy 1 : Targeting labour reserves

First, home-care services can provide job opportunities for the long-term unemployed, the migrant population and adults with disabilities. Targeting the migrant population and adults with disabilities deserves special attention. In some European countries, a substantial number of migrants already have relevant work experience in the informal care sector. Deployment of disabled adults as "hands-on" experts in home care has added value because of the possibilities of identification and empathy with service users.

Second, reaching different groups of labour reserves requires a specific, tailored, target-group approach.

Third, participation in employment programmes has to be free of charge for unemployed job-seekers, and they have to be able to keep any other subsidies or benefits. Financial incentives can encourage them to participate in the programmes.

Fourth, an adequate selection procedure contributes to the success of employment programmes for unemployed job-seekers. Commitment and willingness to work in the home-care sector could be considered as equally important criteria for selection as formal qualifications. Any language barriers can and have to be removed by prequalification training.

Fifth, potential employees have to be selected carefully, but so do their future employers; there has to be a good match between the supply and demand sides of the labour market.

Sixth, the results of vocational training of unemployed job-seekers can be secured and enhanced by quality measures (using officially regulated, approved curricula and quality comparisons between educational institutes) and the proper organisation of training (geographically close to the participants, practice-based and including work placements).

Seventh, a job guarantee beforehand is highly recommended. This will encourage participants to complete the training course, and also means that the training can be fine—tuned to the wishes and needs of the employer.

Eighth, to promote broader employability, vocational training participants should preferably carry out work placements in various branches of the sector.

Ninth, the gaining of work experience by already qualified unemployed job-seekers enhances their chances on the labour market.

Tenth, if necessary, unemployed job-seekers-having successfully finished a job programme—must be supported in finding and keeping a job through the provision of mediation services and follow-up support. Labour cost subsidies can induce employers to employ them.

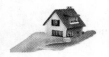

(2) Strategy 2 : Promoting and facilitating education

First, campaigns to encourage young people to consider a career in the care sector are more successful if targeted at specific groups. In this respect, using role models from these groups has added value. There is still much to be done to persuade boys especially that care work is a valid career choice. Such campaigns should have a structured and ongoing character; annual "days" or "weeks" should be connected to activities all year round. In this respect, professional orientation courses in particular-organised by local or regional networks, following a peer-learning approach and including internships in care facilities-are an effective tool.

Second, the content and organisation of health and social care education (including trainee posts) have to be attractive to the students involved, but at the same time suited to the wishes and needs of their future employers. This means there should be an emphasis on practical experience, on-the-job training, intensive coaching and individual attention. Especially beneficial for underprivileged students, such as those with lower educational levels and migrants, is mentoring by teachers or care workers.

Third, trainee posts bridge the gap between care education and the labour market. For less well-qualified students, community-based practical training-in which students are matched by a "labour broker" with local residents that they can help-is a good approach.

Fourth, besides doing work placements as part of their studies, professional apprenticeships for higher-level graduates complement and enhance their professional skills and facilitate integration into the social care labour market. To discourage abuses of professional apprenticeships by employers, subsidies should not be too generous.

(3) Strategy 3: Improving the circumstances of current employees

First, in order to close the gap between supply and demand for jobs in care and support services, improvement of working conditions and terms of employment must have the permanent attention of the social partners and other parties involved.

Second, the professionalisation of the community-based care sector demands the development and enhancement of standards for work and workers in the sector. To adequately implement these standards at regional and local level, it is helpful to establish and maintain partnerships of public and private parties that are responsible for developing, planning, monitoring and evaluating training across the whole home-care workforce. Current care workers can be trained for additional management tasks.

Third, training or retraining employees should ideally be geographically close to the participants, free of charge with

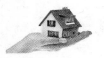

reimbursement of travelling costs and other expenses, and delivered during working hours. It is also more effective and attractive when it is practice-oriented and delivered in venues with modern equipment by skilled guest teachers with a wealth of practical experience. Small class sizes are important, as are regular evaluations and continuous adaptation of the courses to the participants' wishes and needs. Training on an intersectoral basis, with participants from different areas of community-based care and professions, contributes to the cross-pollination of ideas and experience and leads to a more integrated approach to community-based care. It also enhances the broader employability of the participants.

Fourth, the absence of employees undergoing training or retraining for lengthy periods can be offset by using a job-rotation system, in which they are temporarily replaced by unemployed people with appropriate qualifications who need to gain work experience.

Fifth, more traditional ways of training employees should be complemented with modern forms of gaining qualifications, in particular professional validation by experience and e-learning. To encourage validation by experience for those with lower qualification levels, this needs to be based more on practical assessments and less on written tests. The provision of professional support to students improves success rates. Tailoring e-learning systems to the sector enhances their acceptance and use.

(4) Strategy 4: Improving operational management and labour productivity

First, function differentiation or job carving may be applied to home-care work, as this contributes to efficiency, decreases the work pressure on employees at higher qualification levels, and enables disadvantaged groups, such as adults with disabilities, to participate in the labour market. At the same time, giving employees more responsibility makes working in the sector more attractive. This can be done by enhancing executive functions with coordination, advisor or directorial tasks; by creating autonomous self-directing teams; and by encouraging self-management, as in cooperative organisations.

Second, there is much scope for development of direct-payment systems, in which the client becomes an employer of personal assistants. Prerequisites for an adequate direct-payment system include fine-tuning it to the specific needs of the beneficiaries, simplifying its administration and ensuring that emergency measures are in place in case personal assistants are unexpectedly unavailable.

Third, acceptance and use of assisted-living technology such as domotics (home automation) and telecare have been improved by

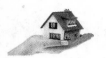

using specialised workers to assess the wishes and needs of potential users. These specialists can also arrange for the installation of the equipment and provide training for users and any others involved.

Fourth, employment services for adults with disabilities, such as sheltered workshops and social enterprises, can improve the quality of life and social inclusion of vulnerable groups. Where possible, sheltered workshop employees should work in the regular labour market, either in disability-friendly or "normal" companies. The deployment of job coaches to support them at work will enhance their functioning in the regular labour market.

Fifth, specialised transport services for adults with disabilities offer a better service when drivers are trained in social care.

3. Policy pointers on sustainability and transferability

First, the sustainability of an initiative deserves particular attention in the case of subsidised projects. After the project period ends, alternative funds have to be found, the coordinating activities of the project management have to be secured and a party to play the leading role must be identified.

Second, the transfer of successful initiatives to other contexts (other regions, countries or sectors) demands a well-thought-out mainstreaming strategy[①]. Such a strategy needs to focus on the receivers of the message (which decision-makers to approach and how); timing the dissemination of the message (when to approach decision-makers); the content of the message (which concrete message to disseminate); the form of the message (which tools to use to deliver the message to decision-makers)[②].

4. General policy pointers

First, each of the various strategies to combat labour market shortages in home-based care has its own merits. Given these complementarities, it should be possible to connect the various measures of the strategies in an integrated approach.

Second, in Europe, the demand for home-based care is expected to increase markedly in the coming years. This will require intensified efforts in labour market policy. Obstacles to the recruitment and retention of personnel in jobs in care and support services that must be addressed include less favourable terms of

---

① Mainstreaming can be defined as embedding successful innovations in regular activities or policies in the same or in other contexts.

② In 2007, Panteia drew up a manual for mainstreaming project results. In 2007, Panteia drew up a manual for mainstreaming project results. See Ministerie van Sociale Zaken en Werkgelegenheid [Netherlands Ministry for Social Affairs] (2007), Verknopen van innovaties. Handleiding voor mainstreaming van projectresultaten [Crosslinking innovations: Manual for mainstreaming of project results], Institute of Policy Research.

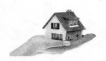

employment (low wages), poor working conditions, long working hours and a negative public image. Aside from national policies, collective agreements reached by social partners can play an important role in tackling these issues.

Third, in some countries, cultural attitudes towards the care of disabled and elderly people have to change. In particular, the idea that family members should be solely responsible for their care at home may limit the ability of those family members to take up paid employment. Increased availability of community-based services contributes to the independence of people with disabilities as well as improving the quality of life of their families.

Fourth, more attention has to be paid to the demand side-clients and institutions. This requires a stock-take of the wishes and needs of clients, and of relevant political developments, given that governments generally determine the budget for the sector.

Fifth, "thinking small" and creating flexibility in projects that operate locally or regionally can help embed new systems into the overall home-care system. This can either be top-down-an adequate translation of large-scale nationwide programmes into regional and local projects—or bottom-up, the nationwide scaling up of successful regional or local pilot projects.

Sixth, the success of labour-market initiatives, especially in the care sector, depends on coordination, cooperation and commitment by the national, regional or local parties involved.

Seventh, "the right person in the right spot" is an important success factor, since the personal characteristics and capacities of the project managers and co-workers involved, and the nature of the personal contacts between them, can make or break initiatives.

Eighth, adequate planning of initiatives is necessary. Progress and results have to be monitored and evaluated. At the same time, however, bureaucracy and administrative burdens have to be avoided as much as possible.

Ninth, the needs of the care sector are increasing, and generating political and public support is essential. Especially in the current economic climate, the importance of the value and needs of the health and social care sector must be communicated clearly to the public. Information and awareness-raising campaigns may be very useful, but they require long-term commitment since it takes time for them to be effective.

Tenth, a very important prerequisite for successful labour market initiatives in this sector is also the availability of sufficient, structural funding.

Eleventh, last but not least, data gathering and use of statistics could be substantially improved to develop, monitor, evaluate and adapt the relevant labour market policies of the national and European authorities.

Bibliography[*]

1. Andor, L. (2011), We Care, How can the EU Care?, Conference Presentation, Social Platform's Annual Conference on Care, 9 December, Brussels.

2. Carretero, S., Stewart, J., Centeno, C., Barbabella, F., Schmidt, A., Lamontagne-Godwin, F. and Lamura, G. (2013), Can Technology-Based Services Support Long-term Care Challenges in Home Care? Analysis of Evidence from Social Innovation Good Practices across the EU, CARICT project summary report, Joint Research Centre of the European Commission, Publications Office of the European Union, Luxembourg.

---

* All Eurofound publications are available at www. eurofound. europa. eu.

3. Cedefop (European Centre for the Development of Vocational Training) (2012), The Role of Qualifications in Governing Occupations and Professions, Cedefop, Thessaloniki.

4. EHMA (European Health Management Association) (2012), EHMA's Workforce Taskforce Discussion Paper: Building a Shared Agenda for Tackling Workforce Challenges, EHMA, Brussels.

5. Eurofound (2006), Employment in Social Care in Europe, Publications Office of the European Union, Luxembourg.

6. European Commission (2006), The Impact of Ageing on Public Expenditure: Projections for the EU25 Member States on Pensions, Health Care, Long-term Care, Education and Unemployment Transfers (2004 – 2050), Special Report No. 1/ 2006, Economic Policy Committee and the Directorate-General of Economic and Financial Affairs, Brussels.

7. European Commission (2007), Health and Long-term Care in the European Union, Special Eurobarometer 283, European Commission, Brussels.

8. European Commission (2010), Second Biennial Report on Social Services of General Interest, SEC(2010) 1284 final, Brussels.

9. European Commission (2010), Europe 2020: A Strategy for Smart, Sustainable and Inclusive Growth, COM (2010) 2020 final, Brussels.

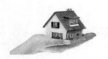

10. European Commission (2011) , The Social Dimension of the Europe 2020 Strategy: A Report of the Social Protection Committee, Publications Office of the European Union, Luxembourg.

11. European Commission (2012) , Commission Staff Working Document on an Action Plan for the EU Health Workforce, SWD (2012) 93 final, Strasbourg.

12. European Commission (2012) , Commission Staff Working Document on Exploiting the Employment Potential of the Personal and Household Services, SWD (2012) 95 final, Strasbourg.

13. European Commission (2012) , Taking Forward the Strategic Implementation Plan of the European Innovation Partnership on Active and Healthy Ageing, COM(2012) 83 final, Brussels.

14. European Commission (2012) , Towards a Job-rich Recovery, COM(2012) 173 final, Brussels.

15. European Commission (2012) , The 2012 Ageing Report: Economic and Budgetary Projections for the 27 EU Member States (2010 – 2060) , European Commission, Brussels.

16. European Commission (2013) , Long-term Care in Ageing Societies—Challenges and Policy Options, SWD (2013) 41 final, Brussels.

17. European Commission (2013) , Social Investment: Commission

Urges Member States to Focus on Growth and Social Cohesion, press release, 20 February.

18. Ewijk, van H., Hens, H., and Lammersen, G. (2002), Mapping of Care Services and the Care Workforce: Consolidated Report, Working Paper No. 3, Thomas Coram Research Unit, Institute of Education, University of London.

19. Genet, N., Boerma, W., Kroneman, M., Hutchinson, A., and Saltman, R. B. (eds.) (2012), Home Care across Europe: Current Structure and Future Challenges, Observatory Studies No. 27, World Health Organization, Copenhagen.

20. Huber, M. (2007), Monitoring Long-term Care in Europe: Background Paper on Care Indicators, European Centre for Social Welfare Policy and Research, Vienna.

21. Korczyk, S. (2004), Long-term Workers in Five Countries: Issues and Options, AARP Public Policy Institute, Washington DC.

22. Lethbridge, J. (2012), Care Home versus Home Care? Which Direction for Care Services in Europe? Eligibility for European Works Councils, EPSU, Brussels.

23. Matrix Insight (2012), EU Level Collaboration on Forecasting Health Workforce Needs, Workforce Planning and Health Workforce Trends—A Feasibility Study, European Commission Executive Agency for Health and Consumers, Luxembourg.

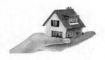

24. Ministerie van Sociale Zaken en Werkgelegenheid [Netherlands Ministry for Social Affairs] (2007), Verknopen van innovaties. Handleiding voor mainstreaming van projectresultaten [Crosslinking innovations: Manual for mainstreaming of project results], Institute of Policy Research.

25. OECD (2011), Health at a Glance 2011-OECD Indicators, OECD Publishing, Paris.

26. OECD (2011), Help Wanted? Providing and Paying for Long-term Care, OECD Publishing, Paris.

27. Panteia, SEOR and Etil (2013), Effectmeting van arbeidsmarktmaatregelen in de zorgsector. Een haalbaarheidsstudie [Effects of labour market measures in the healthcare sector: A feasibility study], Panteia, Zoetermeer, the Netherlands.

28. Rodrigues, R., Huber, M. and Lamura, G. (eds.) (2012), Facts and Figures on Healthy Ageing and Long-term Care, European Centre for Social Welfare Policy and Research, Vienna.

Annex 1 : Analytical Framework

In this book three models were used to provide an analytical framework: (1) the labour market model maps the current and expected situation in demand and supply of labour and identifies discrepancies between demand and supply; (2) a PESTLE analysis describes the external factors influencing the labour market; (3) a solutions model classifies measures to resolve the problems on the labour market.

These models formed the basis for formulating specific research questions, collecting and analysing data and reporting the findings.

1. Labour market model

The key objective of labour market policy is to find a balance

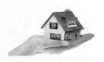

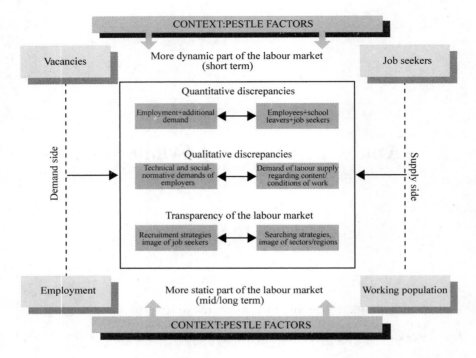

Figure A1 **Labour market model in the context of the PESTLE factors**

Source: Panteia.

between demand and supply. If the demand cannot be satisfied, the potential of a sector is not realised. If there is too much labour available, people will end up in unsuitable jobs or become unemployed. The ideal situation is to have a dynamic balance whereby potential changes and developments in the sector can be accommodated, creating a flexible but sustainable system. Many sectors and countries are faced with a mismatch between supply and demand in their labour markets. This report deals with the very specific situation of community-based care where this mismatch is common and likely to become more marked because of the demographic changes underway. Such labour market discrepancies can be of a quantitative or a qualitative nature, and can be attributed to lack of transparency in the way the labour market is organised. Weighing up demand and supply against one another can indicate where the discrepancies lie.

2. PESTLE analysis

External factors influence the development of the labour market. These factors may pose challenges or create solutions for labour market management. Developments can be identified by looking at six specific dimensions, the basis of a PESTLE analysis.

The six dimensions are the political, economic, social, technological, legal and environmental dimensions. The PESTLE analysis was originally a business-study model to describe a framework of relevant factors at the macro level, used mainly for analysing the business environment of organisations. It is a means of measuring strengths and weaknesses against external factors and can help organisations develop strategies. In the same way, a PESTLE analysis can also be used for a contextual analysis of sectoral labour markets.

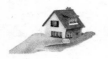

These six dimensions can greatly influence the sectoral labour market, although some are obviously more important than others. In the context of the research questions, particular consideration must be given to the political and economic dimensions, as these have direct effect on the possibility of creating attractive and useful jobs in the community-based care sector. The financial dimension is of special importance here since this is not a generic commercial sector, but one generally financed with public money.

Since the situation in a number of different countries is examined in this report, the labour market discrepancy model connected to the PESTLE factors can help quickly identify where the issues lie in each country. The model provides, in a sense, a common language that describes the challenges faced by the different actors. As previous research has already shown that there is a general shortage of labour in the sector, and in some cases a shortage of jobs, it is to be expected that there are clear discrepancies. The model can swiftly record whether these are qualitative or quantitative, due to a lack of influx into the sector or too great an outflow than can be compensated for, or whether they are triggered by developments in one of the PESTLE dimensions. At the same time, the model offers a structured means of comparison.

3. Solutions model

The PESTLE model bridges the gap between challenges and solutions and so leads to the core objective of this research, namely identifying the instruments that can be employed to recruit and retain workers who will deliver community-based care services.

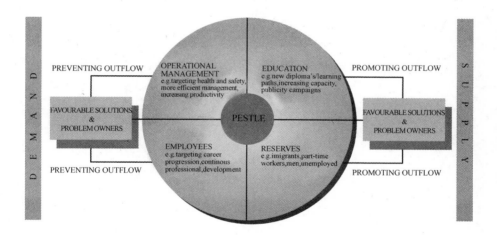

Figure A2 Solutions model

Source: Panteia.

By distinguishing between instruments that stimulate the supply of labour and instruments that temper the demand for labour, it is possible to categorise potential solutions. This leads to the identification of four strategies: (1) targeting labour reserves to

279

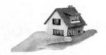

attract new employees to the sector; (2) stimulating and facilitating education for potential employees; (3) improving the situation of current employees to optimise their potential as well as prevent them from leaving the sector; (4) improving the operational management and labour productivity of organisations in the sector.

Most of the instruments already identified in previous research can be located within one of these quadrants. There may also be instruments which aim specifically to alleviate negative pressure from one of the PESTLE factors.

Annex 2 : National Experts

The country and case studies in the framework of this research have been carried out by national experts from the European Network for Social and Economic Research (ENSR), under the supervision of Panteia. On the basis of their input, Panteia drew up this overview report.

The ENSR is a network of institutes specialised in applied social and economic policy research, founded in 1991 by EIM Business & Policy Research (nowadays part of Panteia). The ENSR network has representatives in all the countries of the EU27, and in Norway, Iceland, Switzerland (also covering Liechtenstein), and candidate country Turkey. In all, the ENSR covers 32 countries.

The following ENSR-experts were involved in this book.

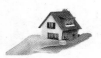

Table A1   **ENSR-experts**

Country	Research institute	Name
Austria	Austrian Institute for SME Research (KMU Forchung)	Ingrid Pecher
Bulgaria	Foundation for Entrepreneurship Development (FED)	Elena Krastenova
Denmark	Oxford Group	Helle Our. Nielsen
France	Centre de. Recherche pour l' Etude et l' Observation des Conditions de Vie (Crédoc)	Isa Aldeghi
Germany	Institut für Mittelstandsforschung (IfM)	Frank Maass, Marina Hoffman
Netherlands	Panteia	Douwe Grijpstra, Peter de Klaver, Jacqueline Snijders, Amber de Graaf, Paul Vroonhof
Poland	Entrepreneurship and Economic Development Research Institute, Academy of Management (EEDRI)	Pawe. Czy.
Portugal	Tecninvest	António Coimbra
Spain	Ikei Research & Consultancy	Jessica Durán
UK	Small Business Research Centre, Kingston University	Eva Kasperova